DEEP SLEEP HYPNOSIS

FALL ASLEEP FAST, SMARTER AND BETTER WITH SELF-HYPNOSIS TECHNIQUES. A MINDFULNESS GUIDE TO SAY STOP ANXIETY, OVERTHINKING AND INSOMNIA

FINN BOLTON

Disclaimer Notice:

Please note the information contained within this document is for educational and entertainment purposes only. All effort has been executed to present accurate, up to date, and reliable, complete information. No warranties of any kind are declared or implied.

Readers acknowledge that the author is not engaging in the endearing of legal, financial, medical, or professional advice. The content within this book has been derived from various sources.

Please consult a licensed professional before attempting any techniques outlined in this book.

By reading this document, the reader agrees that under no circumstances is the author responsible for any losses, direct or indirect, which are incurred as a result of the use of the information contained within this document, including, but not limited to, — errors, omissions, or inaccuracies.

Introduction

Although you might be tired, you may still struggle to actually fall asleep because you aren't able to become fully relaxed. Going to bed doesn't mean just jumping under the covers and closing your eyes. You will also want to ensure that you are keeping up with incorporating relaxation techniques into your bedtime routine so you can stay better focused on getting a complete rest, not one that is constantly disturbed by anxious thoughts.

The following meditation is good for anyone who is about to go to bed. You will want to include this for getting a night of deep sleep, or one that will last for several hours. Keep your eyes closed, and ensure the lighting is right so that there is nothing that will distract you from falling asleep. No lighting is best, but if you do prefer to have some sort of light on, ensure that it is soft yellow or purple/pink. Always choose small lights and nightlights instead of overhead lighting.

Better Sleep Guided Hypnosis

You are in a completely relaxed place, ready to start the process of falling asleep. You are able to stretch your body out, feeling no strain in any limb, muscle, or joint. You are not holding onto any stress within your body. Your eyes are closed, and there is nothing that you need to be worried about in this present moment. You have given yourself permission to fall asleep. You are allowing yourself to take time to relax. You have granted your soul the ability to become completely at ease before falling asleep.

Become aware of your breathing now. Feel how the air moves in and out of you without any effort on your part. Every move that you make is one that helps you to bring in clean, healthy air. In everything that you do throughout the day, your lungs are always working hard to push you through. Everything that requires more strain means making your lungs work harder. Now, we are going to give them a bit of rest, as well. They can never fully stop, but we are going to give them the long, deep, clean, and relaxing breaths that they need now.

Counting while you breathe will help you to become even more relaxed. Breathe in for one, two, three, four, and five. Breathe out for six, seven, eight, nine, and ten.

Once more, this time breathing in through your nose and out through your mouth. Breathe in for ten, nine, eight, seven, six, and out for five, four, three, two, and one.

You are feeling refreshed. You are focused. You are centered. You are at peace.

As thoughts pass into your head, allow them to simply float away. When you think of something that does not pertain to this moment, simply push the thought away. Imagine that you are in a pool and a bug is on the surface of the water. What would you do? At the very least, you would push it away. Gently push your thoughts in another direction and allow them to float away.

Think of your thoughts as if they were sheep jumping over a fence. Imagine them escaping from the pasture in which they are held, only to jump away and go somewhere unknown. Watch as your thoughts hop over the fence. They are passing from your mind out into the world. You are simply releasing them, doing nothing more.

Your thoughts are the stars burning brightly above. They are scary, they are beautiful, and they will always eventually burn out. You will never rid yourself of your thoughts. They will always be dotting the sky. They are so distant, however. They are slow burning. Do not reach for the stars, simply let them be. Let your thoughts slowly burn out now. You only need to be focused on relaxing and becoming more and more at peace.

Feel how you are becoming more and more relaxed. You are letting go of tension in every part of your body. You are becoming more and more focused on centering yourself. You are becoming closer and closer to sleep. You are getting this rest to prepare for the day tomorrow. What happens tomorrow will happen then. There is nothing that you can do about it now. Worrying and stressing isn't going to help you whatsoever. What will help you the most at this moment is drifting deeply into a heavy sleep. Give your body the rest that it needs.

The earth is all asleep now as well. Don't just feel how you are becoming more relaxed. Feel the way that the earth has been tucked into bed as well. Feel how it is now dark and how others are sleeping restfully just as you are. There are some just waking, and some still awake, but they will eventually rest just as you are now. It is time for you to become a part of this whole peaceful earth.

Nothing about the future is scary. You have survived thus far. You are not worried about what is going to happen tomorrow, or the day after, or the day after. Even the bad things that might happen will eventually fade just as well. Nothing is going to keep you from sleeping at this moment. No amount of anxiety will keep you awake.

Everything tomorrow will be unknown. You can prepare but never predict. You are prepared. The best way to ensure that it will be a good day is to get some rest. Allow yourself to get this sleep. Give yourself permission to enjoy this deep and heavy sleep as it exists at this moment.

You are completely comfortable, all throughout your body. You feel relaxation everywhere and you exude peace and serenity.

You are feeling more and more relaxed from the top of your head to the bottom of your toes. You feel your mind start to fade into a dreamlike state. You are feeling as though there is nothing that will keep you awake.

Feel your jawline relax. You hold onto so much tension that you don't even realize. Not now. Not at this moment. You are releasing yourself from all physical strain.

Allow your ears and forehead to be as still and as relaxed as possible. These are heavy and can hold a ton of tension. At this moment, you are letting them become as relaxed as possible. Nothing is going to keep the muscles in your head so tense.

Be aware of the way that we hold our muscles throughout the rest of our bodies. Allow yourself to become relaxed. And even further. And even further. Even when we try to relax, we don't

let go of our bodies all of the ways. Give yourself to rest. Devot
yourself to sleep. Marry the idea of being peaceful.

Allow every bone to become still, relaxed, and serene. You ar
tranquil from the inside out. You are rested from the outside ir

Let your shoulders relax as much as possible. Feel how the
become heavy on your pillow. Your shoulders can hold th
weight of the world. It can feel like everything in your body i
pressing onto them. Let these shoulders drop deeper an
deeper, further and further.

Let your hips be relaxed as well. Your waist, your abdomen—
all of this will also hold tension. Release those feelings. Let you
body become calm and still. Allow yourself to be relaxed all ove
your entire body.

Feel the calm spread from your mind down all the way to you
toes. The peace is like butter, you are the warm toast. Spread i
throughout and allow it to melt into you. Let your body fad
away, slowly becoming more and more peaceful.

Feel your stomach rise as you are breathing. You are breathin
slower and slower, keeping your heart rate low as well. This wil
make it easier to fall into a deep and healthy sleep.

You are becoming more and more relaxed. You are starting to
feel your body become completely calm. Not one single part o
you is still holding onto any tension.

Nothing about the past or the future scares you.

It is time now to fall asleep.

You are going to get the deepest sleep by letting everything go. You are not carrying any fear, anxiety, stress, or pain. You are at peace. You are content. You are calm. You are complete. You are tranquil.

Don't allow thoughts to keep you at the surface of your sleep. Become more and more tired, getting closer and closer to falling all the way asleep.

We are going to count down from ten. When we reach one, you will be fast asleep.

Ten, nine, eight, seven, six, five, four, three, two, one.

Chapter 1 Stages of Sleep

First of all, don't think of sleep as a time when your body "shuts down". Think of it as an active physiological process that kicks off as soon as you shut your eyes and go into sub-consciousness. The first thing that happens when you go into sleep is a dip in the metabolism rate. Other than that, all major organs continue to function with no disruption in their working. The intensity with which the organs work depends on the type of sleep you're in.

There are two types of sleep, Rapid Eye Movement (REM) sleep and non-REM sleep. Scientists have developed clear links to body issues by studying patients' brain activity through a special machine, EEG.

NREM Sleep

Non-Rapid Eye Movement sleep is a type of sleep that is highlighted by reduction in physiological activity. As the duration of sleep increases, the breathing & heart rate go down while the blood pressure drop. This type consists of four stages.

i. Stage 1 – this may be thought of as a hybrid stage when your body is make transition from being awake to going asleep. Brain waves start to slow down while there may be muscle contractions in different part of the body.

ii. Stage 2 – this is a period of light sleep and starts off when eye movements come to a halt. Brain waves become slower generally, except for a few infrequent bursts called sleep spindles. The muscles go into relaxation and body temperature drops.

iii. Stages 3 & 4 – together, these stages are called slow wave sleep and are filled with special types of brain waves called delta waves. The blood pressure falls considerably, the temperature even lower while the breathing slows down. The body becomes completely immobile.

The muscles do have their ability to function but due to the absence of eye movement, it is nearly impossible. When people are woken up at this particular stage of their sleep, they may feel tired and disoriented for a couple of minutes before they normalize. It is also at this very stage that many people experience night terrors and sleepwalking.

REM Sleep

This is the second type of sleep which is marked by serious brain activity. Brain waves come in a desynchronized manner that are similar to those generated when a person is awake. Breathing is rapid and changes rate spontaneously while eyes move randomly in all directions. Limb muscles go into a temporary paralyzed state while the heart rate rises. This is the sleep stage in which dreams occur.

By the looks of it, you may think of REM sleep as the villain but striking the right balance between the two types of sleep is very much necessary for a healthy lifestyle.

During a normal sleeping schedule, the body alternates between REM and NREM stages at night. The pattern is predictable through the use of sensors. A complete sleep cycle consists of NREM and REM stages that change position every 90 – 110 minutes. They must alternate at least 4 times in a night or symptoms of sleep deprivation start kicking in during the waking time period.

Adults spend more than half of their total sleeping time in Stage 2 sleep, 20% in REM sleep and the remaining in all the other stages. The amount of time spent in each stage isn't constant and sometimes shows awkward behavior. As we go deep into the night. The REM period increases while the relaxing portion decreases. By morning all sleep is either REM, or non-REM stage 1 & 2.

With that being said, you are now ready to get a solid picture of how much sleep is necessary for keeping the balance intact. Take a look at the following table:

Age	Sleeping Time
Newborns i.e. 0 - 2 months	12 - 18 hours
Infants i.e. 3 - 11 months	14 - 15 hours
Toddlers i.e. 1 - 3 years	12 - 14 hours
Pre-school children i.e. 3 - 5 years	11 - 13 hours

School-age children i.e. 5 - 10 years   10 - 11
hours

Teens i.e. 10 - 17 years   8 - 9
hours

Adults i.e. 18 +   7 - 9
hours

Sleep Disorders

There are several sleeping disorders that may be working independently or in conjunction to disrupt your sleeping patterns. Here are the most notorious ones:

Insomnia

Insomnia is the most encountered sleeping disorder on the planet, therefore it has to be discussed in depth.

Have you tried going off to bed with the soul intention of dozing off, only to find yourself staring at the ceiling for hours? Next, you even try some of the common methods to bring back sleep like reading a book, but all goes into vain? Even when sleep does come, it's very unrefreshing and you often wake up feeling lethargic? Well, even if one of the answers is yes to the questions then you may be suffering from insomnia.

Insomnia is a common problem especially in today's world where sleeping patterns are intentionally manipulated just so that you can spend more time at work, with your friends or being "productive". Here is a comprehensive list of signs & symptoms associated with insomnia:

-     Rousing up straight in the middle of the night,

-     Having difficulty falling asleep,

-     Going to bed late, but waking up quite early,

-     Restlessness even after sleeping the prescribed amount,

-     Feeling lethargic throughout the day,

-     Loss of appetite,

-     Nausea,
-     Depression & anxiety packed hours,

-     Difficulty in concentrating on everyday problems,

-     Frequent headaches,

-     *Greater error percentage in work,*

Basing the classification on frequency patterns, there are 3 types of insomnia.

-     Acute Insomnia: *Also known as stress induced insomnia, acute insomnia occurs when the disturbances that keep you up at nights or disrupt your sleep last less than 30 days. This type of insomnia is usually caused by a hectic work routine.*

-     Chronic Insomnia: *Unlike acute insomnia, chronic insomnia lasts for more than a month. A longer duration means far reaching effects on a person's lifestyle and therefore, chronic insomnia harms the person both physically as well as psychologically.*

- Transient Insomnia: *This is one of the most common types of insomnia and is triggered by events like traveling to different time zones; it usually lasts for less than a week.*

Insomnia will have a profound impact on your personal life while your

work life will suffer as well. Some of the effects are:

- Reduced cognitive skills,

- Lowered work performance,

- A higher risk of accidents,

- Lagged reaction time,

- Lack of maturity in the immune system,

- Obesity,

- Increased chances of high-risk diseases,

- *Disturbance in social life,*

Sleep Apnea

Also called sleep-disordered breathing, sleep apnea is characterized by brief episodes of shallow breathing. This happens as a result of blockage of the upper airway when the soft tissue in the throat collapses either partially or completely. The blockage comes only for a little while and usually lasts for 10 – 120 seconds. However, the episodes may recur 20 – 30 times in every sleeping hour.

Having sleep apnea means that air flow between your lungs and mouth is not enough, even though breathing continues. As a result of this condition, the amount of oxygen in your blood can dip. This triggers an automatic response from the brain forcing you to wake up just enough so that your airway muscles are back in their normal position. Your body then returns to normal, but the shock caused by the sudden trigger interrupts up the sleeping cycle and resets the stage you were in.

It is known that people who have sleep apnea also snore loudly however this is not always true. Because of the frequent interruptions and switchover from deep sleep to lighter sleep, the mind barely spends any time in restorative sleep, thus the next morning feelings of restlessness and mood swings will surround you.

The following factors may increase your chances of suffering from Sleep Apnea.

- Your throat & tongue muscles relax more than they should,

- Enlarged adenoids and tonsils,

- Head and neck shape that creates a smaller passageway in the mouth,

- Obesity,
- Congestion due to allergies,

Restless Legs Syndrome

RLS is an unpleasant tingling feeling in the legs that can result in mild to severe irritation and lack of deep sleep. People who go through RLS always feel a need to move their legs to get rid of the feeling and as a result find it difficult to go to sleep. Either one or both the legs may be affected by this.

Restless Leg Syndrome is not exclusive to the time when you are trying to sleep but can also occur during times of extended idleness. During sleep RLS results in brief leg movements every 5 – 90 seconds. Sometimes, the movement can be so intense that you may actually wake up.

RLS effects 5 – 15 percent of people in the USA and its occurrence increases as a person ages. RLS itself is a cause of insomnia and is either a result of inheritance or due to improper diet and unhealthy lifestyle. It can be treated quite easily through shifting to a nutritious diet plan, one explained later in the book.

Narcolepsy

If you wait and think about this condition for a second, then this is one of the worst things that can happen to your daily life. During narcolepsy a person suffers from overwhelming daytime sleepiness even after sleeping 8 hours at night. People having narcolepsy often take naps while watching TV or when at work. This can result in lack of concentration, stress and a continuous, bad mood.

People having narcolepsy experience sudden sleep attacks that can last from a few seconds to an hour. During this time, they feel dizziness and the extreme need to sleep. These can be exceptionally disastrous if you're in a meeting because you'll feel as if all control has been transferred to your brain.

It has been found that people having narcolepsy fall directly into REM dream sleep rather than slowly making the shift from non-REM sleep. Narcolepsy isn't a disease, it's a disorder. But even for a disorder it's quite widespread and is almost as common as cystic fibrosis or Parkinson's disease.

You can cure narcolepsy either through drugs or through highly dedicated changes each time you're brain triggers a sleep attack.

Parasomnias

Usually the transition from one sleep state to the next is quite fluid. However, if this transition takes a few bumps then the person asleep may go through bizarre events which may arouse him/her during sleep, called parasomnias. These arousals include events like sleepwalking, bedwetting, night terrors, etc. And even though by the looks of it they may seem common to children, they are reported in adults as well.

The events may be followed by large pupils, agitation and sweating. Children usually outgrow this disorder however one major event that may last even when you're an adult is REM sleep behavior disorder. This is characterized by violent behaviors at night that mostly occur at random. REM sleep is usually followed by a temporary muscle paralysis however when this condition kicks in, the paralysis is lifted. The person may wildly swing one of his limbs, injuring either himself or a bed partner.

Another parasomnia episode that may last is sleep-related eating disorder which means that the person may fall asleep during eating. The problem will not only cause a few mental issues but also a string of digestive conditions as well.

Chapter 2 Build Your Own Self-Hypnosis Script

When you are doing self-hypnosis, there are many different intentions you may have. For that reason, providing you with single script may not be beneficial to assist you in creating you desired results. Instead, we will teach you how you can build your own self-hypnosis script so that you can begin achieving your desired results right away. This structure is to help you build a great personalized script that will specifically target any problem you may be facing and help you gain complete recover from that problem.

Your Induction

Your induction is the part of your script whereby you begin your self-hypnosis. For this part, you want to remind yourself to get comfortable and relax completely. Remind yourself that you need to be in a comfortable position physically so that you can embody all of the benefits of your self-hypnosis. Remind yourself to keep your eyes open at this point and gently gaze at a point directly in front of you.

You can allow yourself to begin paying attention to this item now and familiarizing yourself with it. Then you can also pay attention to what you hear, feel, taste, and smell. As you notice each thing, allow yourself to "explore" it with your mind for a few moments before pushing the thought away. This will help you ignore it later on, and it also helps activate your mind's eye

Once you are done exploring with your senses, remind yourself to close your eyes and go deeper into a state of relaxation.

Your Deepening Technique

The easiest deepening technique starts with your breath. That is, you want to notice that with each breath you take, you become more relaxed. You may state that you are simply going to relax more, or you may create an opportunity whereby each breath feels like you are inhaling relaxation and exhaling tension and stress.

Affirm how wonderful it feels to be so relaxed and allow yourself to sit with this great feeling for some time before moving on to do a body scan, as outlined in Then, imagine that you are going down a flight of stairs. Each step you go down takes you deeper into a state of relaxation until you reach the bottom of the stairs. There, you are faced with a door. When you enter that door, you will be in a complete state of relaxation whereby you can begin your hypnosis intentions.

Programming Exercises

Programming exercises are ones that you can use to help you see your desired results. You can guide yourself through a visualization that you can pre-create before entering your hypnotic state, or you can use affirmations.

If you are using visualization, you want to generate a visualization whereby you will be overcoming your challenge, and it feels genuinely good. Notice what it looks and feels like to overcome your challenge and notice all of the feelings you get as a result. Be sure to regularly affirm yourself and your success.

If you are using affirmations, choose two or three affirmations beforehand that you will use when you are in your hypnotic state to achieve your desired results. Then, you can cycle through these over and over once you are in your deeply relaxed state.

You can also combine these two practices for a stronger script and stronger results.

Exit Strategy

Your exit strategy is where you begin to take yourself out of your hypnotic state so that you can "come back to the room." A great way to do this is to count from one to five and let yourself awaken more and more with each count. Each count allows you to feel the energy flowing into your body, awakening you from your state of relaxation. You can imagine that each number takes you through the five major parts of your body: your arms, legs, torso, head, and then your eyes open.

Chapter 3 Deeper Sleep Hypnosis

What is the best position to sleep? Well, that is going to be up to what is the most comfortable pose for you when it comes to slumbering in bed. Anyone who is going to be doing this deep-sleep meditation needs to get into the most comfortable position. Think of it as if you are getting ready to snooze for the night.

Being in a position that is not going to bring you the most comfort will only defeat the purpose of the guide and will not allow you to meditate effectively.

These hypnotic practices should be done at night when you are about to go to bed. Do not do them for the first time if you are planning to, say, go shopping or ride a plane or a bus. Even though these are times when you might wish to fall asleep, you never know how your body might react.

Before-Bed Hypnosis

Be sure to darken your room until it is pitch-black. Close the blackout blinds or cover the windows with dark-colored fabrics. Make sure that there are absolutely no distractions that can prevent you from making the most out of this hypnosis. Play the sounds that you find comforting as well, preferably the ones with isochoric tones to remain focused.

If you have an essential oil diffuser, you should set it up before lying down as well. In case you do not own one, then apply the essential or aromatic oil of your choice on your temples or wrists. Nevertheless, you can do away without such oils, too. They are merely optional tools that may help you ascertain that you are ready to start the hypnosis before bed and that you are well-prepared to do it.

Once all of that is done, the next thing that you want to do is make sure that you end up in a comfortable position. This way, you can genuinely get into a state of relaxation so that you will be able to get into a deep sleep.

This hypnosis is going to guide you on how to feel completely rested before your bedtime. You are going to let go of the distractions of the day and feel yourself be more peaceful than ever. It is going to start with you focusing on your breathing and doing a rhythmic count to get you into the hypnotic mode. So, first, ensure that you are breathing deeply, feeling it all the way inside your body, and letting the entire breath come out before starting again.

Too often, we will find that we are taking short breaths, which only keep us anxious and alert. We are going to guide you into drawing in a long and deep breath while relaxing your body to help snap you into this hypnosis. We are going to count down from 20; when we reach one, you will already be in a relaxed state. Afterward, we will help you to visualize the perfect scenario to prepare for bed and fall into a deep sleep.

As I count, breathe in slowly from 20 to 11, and then breath out from ten to one. Continue to do this kind of deep breathing until you reach a point in which your body feels extremely calm.

Breathe in for twenty, nineteen, eighteen, seventeen, sixteen, fifteen, fourteen, thirteen, twelve, eleven, and now out for ten, nine, eight, seven, six, five, four, three, two, one. You are now in a trance, and nothing else is coming into your mind.

You feel yourself in a state of deep relaxation. You are not concerned with the things that have been bothering you throughout the day.

Imagine that you are on a beach. Your feet are nestled in the white sand, and nothing around you attracts too much of your attention. Instead, you are focused on feeling as good as possible as you are on this beach.

As people walk by along the shore, you do not feel the need to look at them. It's not because you do not care about others. You're simply not concerned with whatever business they have on the same beach. Now, you watch them slowly get closer to you, and then they fade into the distance as they walk away.

The people passing you on the beach are much like the thoughts that keep you up at night. They are intrusive. They come out of nowhere. You might think of something that happened ten years ago or earlier that day that embarrassed you as well. As similar ideas come into your head, you allow it to fade away into oblivion.

Nonetheless, you should know that these thoughts will always be there. There is no getting rid of them entirely. Each time something drifts into your mind to keep you awake, though, you merely have to let it pass by slowly.

The only thing that you can hear is the sound of the waves in the water. They slap onto the shore and continue to emerge one after another. These waves can be powerful, but they are bringing you a plethora of peace and serenity.

They continue to wash along the shore just as if you are washing your brain of the day. We shower to keep our hair and skin clean, but what are we doing to rid our brains of filth and grime

The sound and thoughts of the waves are coming one after another, each new wave taking something from the shore and swallowing it back into the ocean.

These waves are taking the thoughts that clutter your mind and washing them away. There are some ideas that need to hang onto, and memories can be important. The thoughts that keep you awake at night, however, serve no purpose.

You are watching the water now as they keep getting sucked up and sent back into the water. There is nothing that concerns you now other than relaxing on the sand.

You feel your body become a part of the ground. Before, it was filled with tension, and you were unable to relax. You could feel the strain in every part of your muscles from the way that your body was keeping itself so tense and tight. You are not concerned with that anymore. The only thing that you have to focus on is making sure that you are as weightless as possible.

You are still on the sand. You are heavy enough to leave an imprint into it, but you are also light because you do not hold anything in your body. The only thing that your muscles are concerned with is supporting the important parts of your body

You are not carrying extra stress, tension, and strain on the internal organs that need to stay healthy to keep functioning. Your bones and muscles are sore and achy from holding onto so much stress, but you are letting that all go now. It is like every negative feeling becomes another grain of sand. You don't need to worry about them anymore.

You are now completely still in the sand, focusing on nothing but the sky. As you are laying on the beach, you can feel the warm sun hit your skin. It is not too hot to the point that it is burning, but it is also keeping you from feeling cold in case the wind blows and hits your body.

You are looking up at the blue sky, noticing how perfectly clear it is. There is nothing for you to concentrate on, so you take in the sky as a whole, as the one thing that it is.

The sky, the sun, and our planet are all important when it comes to sustaining life. Trees and flowers grow desperately to reach the sun, and you know how powerful it can be. You feel its warmth kiss you, but it does not keep you awake. It fills the sky, but that doesn't mean that it keeps you alert. Instead, you tend to relax when you see how serene the sky can be.

You are now noticing that the sky is slowly fading to black, and it becomes more and more difficult to keep your eyes open. As we count down from twenty again, you will be able to rest well, ready to fall into a deep sleep. You can either drift off completely afterward or carry on to other meditations to help you fade away. Again, breathe in for the first ten counts, and out for the final ten counts.

Breathe in for twenty, nineteen, eighteen, seventeen, sixteen, fifteen, fourteen, thirteen, twelve, eleven, and now out for ten, nine, eight, seven, six, five, four, three, two, one.

Relaxation Hypnosis for Deep Sleep

For this exercise, make sure that you have the background set up perfectly. Turn on some music and fill the room with fragrances from the essential oils, considering you have chosen to use those tools to aid you with the hypnosis.

Your room is pitch-black, and you have no distractions around you that can prevent you from going into a deep sleep. You should be physically comfortable as well; otherwise, the hypnosis won't be effective. You may still fall asleep, and the meditation may work for you, but you will end up waking up feeling extremely sore and out of sorts if you have not taken care of your physical comfort before preparing for bed. Thus, as previously mentioned, you should look for a pose that will make you feel relaxed night after night. If you are unsure of which sleeping position is the best for you, then you will need to experiment with that in your own time.

Now, I am going to guide you into taking a long and deep breath as you try to loosen up your body. This will allow you to snap into a hypnotic trance. We are going to count down from 20. Once we reach one, you will be in a completely relaxed state. We will then help you visualize the perfect scenario to fall into a deep sleep.

As I count, breathe in slowly from 20 to 11, and then breath out from ten to one. Continue to do this kind of deep breathing until you feel that you have reached total relaxation.

Breathe in for twenty, nineteen, eighteen, seventeen, sixteen, fifteen, fourteen, thirteen, twelve, eleven, and now out for ten, nine, eight, seven, six, five, four, three, two, one. You are now in a relaxed trance, and nothing is coming into your mind.

Your eyes are deeply closed, and you do not feel bothered by anything. You are resting well, and you sense the basic soreness of the day leave your body.

You start to feel the muscles in your shoulders ease. Your hips and back are comfortably pressed on the mattress as well. With your eyes still closed, your lids are becoming heavier and heavier. The dark and peaceful ambiance is helping you to feel comfortable and ready to drift off. You are not afraid of anything right now.

Your room may always be dark, but it may only bring you fear. Night after night, you cannot rest as much as you need. It can feel as if you will never catch up sometimes, too. However, with these meditations, you will be able to get back to a place where you can go into a deep slumber every night.

As you start to slip into a different state of consciousness, imagine walking into a dark and almost empty room. The only thing that exists in this space is a long, soft mattress. On top of it are several pillows and blankets, all of which you can choose from. You walk towards the bed and observe the pillows for a

31

moment, but you realize that rather than taking one and using that, you are going to take everything.

You spread the pillows across the mattress and let yourself slide under the covers slowly. The door is closed behind you - locked, in fact - and there isn't a soul around to bother you. In some situations, such a peaceful ambiance might actually frighten you, but the only thing that you should care about right now is getting to sleep. You are completely at ease in this room and not holding onto any fear whatsoever.

As you lay on the bed, allow yourself to stretch out. You tuck the pillows perfectly behind your head, and your feet have plenty of room to breathe. You don't have anyone to share the bed with, but you are not lonely. You are simply focused on getting the best sleep of your life.

In the past, it has been hard to fall asleep for you. Once you do, though, it is equally difficult to stay asleep. Now, you understand that the problem is that you do not feel relaxed enough. You will wake up again if you let the anxious thoughts remain in your mind. If your body is not comfortable, it will cause you to stir as well.

You stretch your leg out, moving it across the bed under the sheets. Then, you feel the coolness of fresh, untouched blanket over your leg. You shift your leg back next to the other for warmth. The cool sheets help to send a soothing sensation throughout your body, making you even more appreciative of the warmth that comes from you. Your arms are stretched out as well, and nothing about the bed makes you feel uncomfortable in any way.

You let the coldness, hunger, sleepiness, heat, and other feelings pass through you and realize that you are not dealing with any of these things right now. You are simply there in the bed, focused on drifting away to sleep.

You feel yourself slipping deeper into a state of relaxation. Nothing else that is going on in the world matters right now. Even if you have an incredibly anxious and pressing matter to deal with, sleep is the only thing that you should be focused on.

Everything will work itself out. Everything has a solution. Everything has a plan. Right now, you should get some sleep. You won't be able to accomplish any task if you are not well-rested.

Allow your mind to push these anxious thoughts out of your head slowly as soon as they start to come in. Don't give into them. Instead, remember to concentrate on falling asleep completely.

Keep on sensing how your body feels to make sure that you are not tensing up, too. Start from the top of your head. Let it fall heavy on the pillow. Keep your facial muscles relaxed and have your neck comfortably supported. Maintain the looseness of your shoulders, chest, and arms as well. Furthermore, let your core melt into the bed so that your abdominal muscles are not stiff. If any part of your body is still taut or you are aching somewhere, then it won't allow your brain to fall asleep. You cannot expect the hypnosis to work without taking this step.

Your eyelids are getting heavier and heavier now. Even though you think that you are already engulfed in nightfall, everything gets just a little bit darker. You can't even hear any birds chirping or other nightly noises at the moment. Those things are still out there, but none of that is going to affect you right now.

This is your world. This is the place that you are supposed to be in. No matter what else is going on in your life, in the world you need to be here right now. You need sleep to survive, to be healthy. If you don't fall into a deep slumber, you can't achieve all the other things that you want to do.

We are going to count down from 20 once more. When we reach one, you will be able to drowse off immediately.

Breathe in for twenty, nineteen, eighteen, seventeen, sixteen, fifteen, fourteen, thirteen, twelve, eleven, and now out for ten, nine, eight, seven, six, five, four, three, two, one. You are now ready to fall asleep.

Chapter 4 Sleep Scripts

Now that you are ready to fall asleep take a deep breath in. Exhale slowly and expel any tension that may have built up during the last few exercises.

As you settle in for sleep, you may begin to have thoughts about what you have done today or things you need to get done tomorrow. Take another deep breath and let those thoughts go with your next exhale. At this moment, all you need to do is clear your mind. Today is over and tomorrow will come whether you worry about it or not. For now, clear your mind so you can wake up strong and healthy for your duties tomorrow.

For now, I want you to draw your attention to your body. Where did you store your tension today? I invite you to focus your attention on the tension and let it go as we practiced earlier. Feel now where your body is relaxed. Take a few moments to appreciate the sense of relaxation your body is feeling at this moment and allow it to spread through your whole body from head to toes.

Before you drift off to bed, let's fill your mind with peaceful images. By promoting positive mental images, this will help you relax and can help avoid nightmares. As we begin, I would like you to visualize a place where you feel safe and comfortable. Take a few moments and imagine how the place would be.

When you have your safe place in mind, I would like you to start to relax your body again. In order to get rid of nightmares, you will need to release all tension from your body. When we are fearful, this can create tension in our body. Try to pay special attention to your shoulders, hands, back, neck, and jaw. Often times, these are areas where our tension can creep in.

If you feel any of these areas tensing up, focus your attention here. Breathe in…and breathe out…choose to relax and soften these areas. As you breathe, imagine the air bringing total relaxation to these areas and allow the tension to leave your body. I invite you to continue this pattern until your breathing becomes deep and slow again.

Notice now how your body has become more relaxed than it was before. Feel as your muscles sink into the bed as you relax further and deeper. Your jaw is becoming loose. Your mouth is resting, and your teeth are slightly apart. Now, your neck is relaxing, and your shoulders are falling away. Allow this to happen and let your muscles become soft.

I want you to return to your safe place. Imagine that this place is spacious, comfortable, and filled with a positive light. In this place, you have nothing to worry about, and you have all the time in the world to focus on yourself.

In this safe place, I want you to imagine the sun streaming in. The light fills you with warm and positive emotion. Thee are windows where you can see the beautiful nature outside. Your space can be wherever you want it to be. It can be by the mountains, by the ocean, or perhaps even on a golf course.

Return your focus back on your safe place. Imagine how warm and comfortable the room is. Walk over toward the comfortable bed and imagine how wonderful it feels to sink into the sheets. The sun is shining down on you, and you feel relaxed and warm.

The bed is so soft around you, and you feel so at peace at this moment.

Notice now how these peaceful thoughts begin to fill your mind. They are filling your conscious and are clear. Any other thoughts you had before are drifting away. Your mind is falling into a positive place as you feel yourself drifting away. The space around you is safe and peaceful, and beautiful.

Any other thoughts you have at this moment, pass through your mind and drift off like clouds drifting by. Allow these thoughts to pass without judgment. There is no sense in dwelling on them when you are in such a safe place. All you have at this moment is peace and quiet.

Any time a worrying thought arises, you turn your focus back to your safe place. In this location, you can get rid of any stress you may have on a daily basis. You are here to relax and enjoy this moment. There is nothing that can bother you. You are free from stress and responsibilities here.

When you are ready, you feel your body begin to drift off to sleep. You are beginning to slip deeper and deeper toward the land of dreams. As you feel your attention drift, you are becoming sleepier, but you chose to focus on counting with me. As we count, you will become more relaxed as each number passes through.

We will now take a few breaths, and then I will count from the number one to the number ten. As you relax, your mind will drift off to a deep and refreshing sleep. Ready?

Breathe in…one…two…three…and out…two…three.

Breathe in…one…two…three…and out…two…three.

Breathe in…one…two…three…and out…two…three.

Wonderful. Now, count slowly with me…one…bring your focus to the number one…

Two…you are feeling more relaxed…you are calm and peaceful…you are drifting deeper and deeper toward a wonderful night of rest.

Three…gently feel as all of the tension leaves your body. There is nothing but total relaxation filling your mind and your body. At this moment, your only focus is on quietly counting numbers with me.

Four…picture the number in your mind's eye. You are feeling even more relaxed and at peace. Your legs and arms are falling pleasantly heavy. You are so relaxed. Your body is ready for sleep.

Five…you are drifting deeper. The sleep begins to wash over you. You are at peace. You are safe. You are warm and comfortable.

Six…so relaxed…drifting off slowly…

Seven…your mind and body are completely at peace. You have not felt this calm in a while…

Eight…everything is pleasant. Your body feels heavy with sleep.

Nine...allow your mind to drift...everything is floating, and relaxing...your eyelids feel comfortable and heavy...your mind giving in to the thought of sleep.

Ten...you are completely relaxed, and at peace...soon, you will be drifting off to a deep and comfortable sleep.

Now that you are ready to sleep, I will now count from the number one to number five. All I want you to do is listen gently to the words I am saying. When I say the number five, you will drift out of hypnosis and sleep comfortably through the night.

In the morning, you will wake up feeling well rested and stress-free. You have worked on many incredible skills during this session. You should be proud of the hard work you have put in. Now, it is time to sleep so you can wake up in the morning feeling refreshed.

Chapter 5 Diet & Sleep

As you already know, sleep deprivation can have seriou harmful effects on your overall health, so helping your body ge a good night sleep is not such a bad idea. How can you do this The first thing you need is to be conscious that not only stres and problems affect your sleep, but your diet also plays a important role in all of this.

If you want to sleep like a baby, if you want to avoid waking u in the middle of the night or having trouble sleeping, you hav to realize and accept that what you eat during the day, especiall in the last few hours before sleeping, affects you.

The food you eat for dinner or in the hours before you go t sleep has a tremendous effect on your sleep. Food can affect th quality and duration of your sleep. This is why it's so importan to eat healthy, especially at dinnertime; eating foods that wor with your body and not against it. If you help yourself with th right foods, I can assure you, you will sleep better every nigh and by doing this you will feel good, more active and reste every day.

There's a direct relation between your eating habits and sleep this is because some nutrients interact with hormones an chemicals that affect your relaxation and sleep. You see hormones are responsible for wakefulness and sleep, and botl states are related to the circadian rhythm. This circadian rhythn can be altered, especially after thirty years of age, by stress, nigh shifts, long intercontinental flights or your diet. Luckily, there' a lot you can do to help your body, and it all starts with a prope diet.

Many people say that to have a good sleep, abundant and heavy dinners should be avoided. This is completely true, but it is also true that you can't go to the other extreme. You should never go to bed on an empty stomach, or eating so little that you wake up in the middle of the night with your stomach growling because you are starving. The ideal is to have a dinner that produces the sensation of satiety but based on nonfat foods and easy digestion.

It's also not recommendable to eat dinner and immediately go to bed; this is related to the accumulation of fat and it does not help in sleep at all. The best is to have dinner and wait an hour and half or two hours before going to bed.

Hormones

Let's talk a little about serotonin and melatonin; these are two chemical substances that play such an important role in sleep balance.

Serotonin is a neurotransmitter that moves information through different parts of your brain. It directly or indirectly controls almost every function of your brain, like your mood, sexual functions and sleep cycles. Serotonin levels in your body are high when you are awake and active, and almost absent when you are in the deepest stage of sleep.

While you are asleep, melatonin levels in your body augment significantly. Melatonin production depends on the pineal gland, which is fed by serotonin. While light augments levels of serotonin, darkness stimulates the production of melatonin. For

41

this reason, the right amounts of serotonin and melatonin have to be present in your body to get a good and profound sleep.

Hormones And Diet

The release of these two neurotransmitters depends on the availability of an amino acid called tryptophan. Despite being an essential substance, tryptophan is not produced naturally in the body. Luckily, this amino acid is present in many foods that can help balance the levels of serotonin and melatonin that directly influence your sleep.

Foods High In Tryptophan

- *Fish, especially blue fish like sardines, mackerel and tuna. Also white fish like cod and halibut.*
- *Red meat*
- *Eggs*
- *Dairy products as cheese and yogurt*
- *Legumes such as lentil, chickpeas, peas, beans and peanuts*
- *Grains such as rice, wheat, oatmeal and corn*
- *Dry fruits such as almonds, pine nuts, pistachio and cashews*
- *Fruits like avocado, orange, dates, blueberries, grapes, apples, strawberries and cherries*
- *Vegetables such as spinach, zucchini, asparagus, celery, lettuce, tomatoes, carrots, cucumber and watercress*

Other Important Nutrients

For the adequate release of these substances, besides tryptophan, Omega 3 and Omega 6 fatty acids are needed. You can find these fatty acids in some fish like sardines, salmon, halibut, and cod or in dry fruits, olive and sunflower oil.

Magnesium is considered by many to be the "anti-stress mineral," and they might be right. Low levels of magnesium can cause sleeping disorders or symptoms that interrupt your sleep. Augmenting your levels of magnesium can help you sleep better at night as well. Nuts, spinach, carrots and peas are rich in magnesium and Vitamin B6, which helps the metabolism of tryptophan. Bananas are like natural sleeping pills, an injection of serotonin and melatonin and rich in magnesium: a natural muscle relaxer.

Calcium helps the brain utilize tryptophan more effectively, so melatonin is produced faster, and this induces sleep and relaxation. A small glass of warm milk can also help a lot for a good night's sleep as well as yogurt.

Some carbs with a low glycemic index can also help you sleep. Glucose levels in the blood inhibit hypocretin, which is a neurotransmitter that keeps you awake. But, remember, measure is the key. If you have a big plate of pasta then the effect will be the complete opposite; your digestion will be slow and your sleep fragmented and not repairing at all. Oatmeal is one of the best sources of melatonin, so keep it in your diet.

Vitamin C, found in oranges and kiwis, helps the body maintain the levels of magnesium active and intervene with the GABA, which is a neurotransmitter that inhibits the central nervous system and is vital for a good night sleep.

An example of a good dinner would be an omelet with zucchini or any vegetables you love, chicken soup or vegetable soup, and a small portion of rice. A plate of salad with tomato, tuna and olive oil are also great choices for dinner. Oatmeal and blueberries, a warm glass of milk and some fruits can also help. Use your imagination; you have plenty of things to choose from that are healthy and will help you sleep like a baby!

What To Avoid

An excessive amount of food for dinner, whether it contains tryptophan or not, is definitely not beneficial for sleep. There are some things you should definitely stay away from; let's check them out.

- *Foods high in fats: these nutrients are the most difficult to digest, so your stomach will still work when you are asleep. Fats make you feel heavy and they are the first thing to avoid.*
- *Sugar: chocolate and candies eliminate somnolence and make you alert, so please stay away from them!*
- *Caffeine drinks such as coffee and tea should be avoided because they are stimulants. If you love coffee drink it at least four or five hours before you go to bed. Now, sodas...forget about them. They are two times worse for your sleep because they contain caffeine and sugar.*
- *A glass of wine can be relaxing for many, but even though it has a sedative effect, it does not produce a repairing sleep. Alcohol dehydrates your body and intervenes with the repairing effects of sleep.*

- *-Avoid drinking liquids in high quantities before you sleep because it will make you get up to go to the bathroom during the night. Stay hydrated during the day, but keep liquids in check at night.*

These are the basics of nutrition and sleep. Try to work with your body; you will feel the difference. And remember that a good night's sleep will not only make you feel fresh and active every day, but also prolong your life and your quality of life.

Chapter 6 Guided Sleep Meditations
Retrace Your Day

In the wake of a difficult day at work, the vast majorit lamentably falls on autopilot, executes an arbitrary arrangemen of undertakings, and inevitably nods off, while it's imperative t unwind in the wake of a monotonous day at work. Your evenin propensities are basic to preparing your psyche and body fo sleep.

Review your day, in detail, action-by-action. Starting from getting up in the morning, through showering and havin breakfast, spend 20-25 seconds on each of the day's event however small. Survey your day and investigate its occasion What went well? What went poorly? What territory would yo be able to become most from beginning tomorrow? What more, by what method will you do this? This spots you in a enabling development outlook.

By looking into and learning, you're developing and advancin at a quick rate, which means you'll arrive at your objective quicker than the normal individual. Completing off you evening schedule with five minutes of day-tracking assists wit tomorrow as well as it causes you get fixated on the presen minute while tending to your inner world. This is a great way t begin powering down, before going to bed.

Locate an agreeable, calm spot to sit or rest

Take your place

You can do this practice sitting or lying down

Stay in completely relaxed manner

Don't do anything immediately

Ground yourself first

Just sit or lie down completely relaxed for a few minutes

Get into a comfortable position

Keep your back straight

Ensure that your shoulders are also straight

Your back and neck should be in a straight line

Now, close your eyes

If you are sitting

Lean slightly forward and then backward

Lean-to your left side and then to your right

Now, bring yourself to the center and find the best and most comfortable position

Feel your head positioned on your neck

Raise your chin slightly upwards

This will help you in placing your focus between your eyebrows

If you are lying down

Ensure that your spine and neck are straight

Keep your palms open facing upwards

Try to feel your whole body

Notice if there is tension anywhere

If you feel any part tense, release the tension

Adjust your body to release the pressure

Begin by taking a few deep breaths

Breathe in

Breathe out

Don't rush the process

Breathe in

And breathe out

Now focus your mind on the day passed watching it like a movie
that replays in your mind

Pay attention to your life reviewing what happened

Try to remember everything

Start with the first thing you remember

What it was to wake you up?

Perhaps, the alarm clock went off

Or the bright light of the sun

Or maybe your pet came to get you out of bed

What did you do as soon as you wake up?

Did you kiss your sweet half?

Probably you got up instantly and went to the bathroom

Or you went to the kitchen to feed your pet

Try to remember every detail as precisely as possible

Note each nuance

What did you have for breakfast?

How was taste, can you feel it in your mouth?

What did you do after?

Perhaps you heard something funny or alarming on the radio as you were driving to work

Obviously, you remember highly emotional times like when you had an argument with someone, but you may not be able to remember anything about how you came home from work.

Don't worry about it

This powerful meditation practice will help you to be more mindful and focus on living your life to the fullest every day

Now look back on your day again

And notice how you acted in the many situations in which you found yourself

Help yourself with one of the following questions:

Did I follow my plans for the day?

What was a highlight on my day?

What didn't go so well?

Where I could have been more effective today?

What could I do better?

Where I could have been more (loving, helpful, kind, focused, calm, patient, determined or any other quality or characteristic you like) today…

What have I learned that can help me tomorrow?

Reply the questions without any judgment or self-criticism

Just observe events from the day appears in your mind

Be honest with yourself

Be sure to notice the context, the details of what happened and how you acted

By doing this you increase focus and clarity in your mind

You train your subconscious to work on fast and logical solutions to the tasks you may face with during the day

If there is some event that bothering your mind

Replay it in your mind the way you would have preferred to have done it had you been more conscious at the time

This exercise influencing your subconscious helps to install a new positive behavior and evoke it the next time you find yourself in a similar situation.

It's time to come back

Become aware of your surrounding

Become aware of your breathing

You are doing great

Notice how clear and calm is your mind now

There is no fear now

There is no stress

No thoughts bothering you

You are completely calm and relaxed

Now you can open your eyes

Or choose to fall asleep.

Wash Away the Pressures of the Day

Showering is something that (nearly) everybody does day by day, as it's a simple to-execute answer for improving your rest. For individuals experiencing a sleeping disorder, a shower or shower can profit by enabling them to unwind and set up the brain and body for bed.

You can make your bath or shower even more relaxing by trying out some simple meditations. It is a practice of using the water as a mechanism to wash away the stress, tension and anxiety within your body. Meditating in the shower can help you find a deeper sense of relaxation and calm. The best reason to try shower meditation is that it does not take any additional time in your day.

Adjust the water pressure and temperature to a warm, soothing and comfortable setting

Begin by focusing on your breath

Inhale slowly and deeply

Feel the cleansing air fill your chest

Now exhale

Letting tension, stress, negative thoughts and negative energy flow away with the air.

Now repeat

Take a deep breath

And slowly exhale through your mouth

Again, breathe in through your nose

Breathe out through your mouth

One more time

Inhale deeply through your nose

And slowly exhale through your mouth

Now face the shower stream

Relax your entire body

Step under the waterfall, allowing the water to run down directly onto the back of your neck

Close your eyes, if it is possible

Take a moment to focus all your attention on how it feels

Allow your mind to quiet for a few moments

Just focus on what you are experiencing

Enjoy the warmth

Continue deep breathing

Notice how the water feels against your skin

Focus on the steady rhythmic drumming of the water

On your neck

On your shoulders

On your arms

On your hands

On your back

On your legs

On your feet

Let your body relax

Allow all the tension to drift away

Notice how the water pulls the weight of the tension down and out of you

Your limbs and body get lighter and lighter

Feel lightness in your body

Now you are very relaxed.

Now step back out of the waterfall

Start to cleanse your body

Take your shower gel or soap and massaging it into your skin

Start at your arms and shoulders and then go down

As you soap yourself

Repeat the following affirmation

"I am cleansing my body and mind to feel calm, peaceful and relaxed"

Keep repeating this affirmation as you scrub your body all over

"I am cleansing my body and mind to feel calm, peaceful and relaxed"

Feel the way the shower gel is cleansing you

"I am cleansing my body and mind to feel calm, peaceful and relaxed"

Again

"I am cleansing my body and mind to feel calm, peaceful and relaxed"

As you rinse off the soap

Imagine these feelings as dirt on your skin that can run down the drain

Feel the water take everything with it.

Next turn to face away from the shower stream

Step backward now, so that you feel the water beat down on the top of your head

Close your eyes, if it is possible

Continue deep breathing

Imagine the water is a dark blue color

Feel the blue water flow slowly down your head

Neck

Shoulders

Arms

Fingertips

Chest

Belly

Back

Thighs

Calves

Toes

And then run down the drain

Visualize the blue water washing away all the tension, strain and anxiety from your head and body

Envision the power of the blue water taking away all your negative thoughts

Feel sadness, fear, regret, anger, and depression washing right off you

Falling into the drain and disappearing

Imagine all your problems are going down the drain leaving you forever

Feel calm and relaxation

Enjoy the clarity of your mind

Allow yourself to remain for a while before you get out of the shower

Just stay enjoying the moment

You are calm

Your mind is clear

Your body is light and relaxed

You are fully relaxed

Now slowly step out of the water stream

And open your eyes.

Have a good night!

Guided Visualization

Guided imagery or perception includes utilizing our creative mind to help put our body in a progressively relaxed state. Similarly, as our body can wind up tense and worried in light of the everyday events that put us or on edge, it can likewise turn out to be progressively quiet and loose in light of calm, serene, and lovely surroundings.

One of the most fundamental approaches to use guided imagery to unwind is to close our eyes and envision being in a spot that is serene and unwinding to us. It teaches us to utilize most of your faculties in our creative mind and appreciate being there for a couple of minutes. We can use this as a customary unwinding exercise or in the midst of stress when you have to unwind.

Here, we are focusing on imagining the positive scenarios and events which make us happy and bring calmness to our stressed mind. Rehearsing this method over some stretch of time causes us to lessen everyday tension, and handle stress in an increasingly quiet and sure way. Practicing this technique each day for at least 10-15 minutes would reduce our stress levels and help bring our sleep cycle on track. We must not fall asleep while the session is going on as it would not be effective, however, we can complete the session and go to sleep.

Locate an agreeable, calm spot to sit or rest

Take your place

It is better lying down into your bed

But you can also choose to do this practice seating

Stay in completely relaxed manner

Don't do anything immediately

Ground yourself first

Just sit or lie down completely relaxed for a few minutes

Get into a comfortable position

Keep your back straight

Ensure that your shoulders are also straight

Your back and neck should be in a straight line

Now, close your eyes

Ensure that your spine and neck are straight

Keep your palms open

Try to feel your whole body

Notice if there is tension anywhere

If you feel any part tense, release the tension

Adjust your body to release the pressure

Begin by taking in a deep breath

And noticing the feeling of air filling your lungs.

Hold your breath for a few seconds.

Breathe out slowly

Letting the tension leave your body.

Make slowly another deep breath

And hold it.

Slowly release the air.

Breathe in slower now,

Hold your breath.

Slowly release the breath

And feel the tension leaving your body.

Continue breathing slowly through all the practice.

Now, imagine that you are lying on a white soft fluffy cloud

High in the sky on a beautiful night

The cloud holds you safely

Floating across the sky

It is moving very slowly

You are floating peacefully and comfortably

Under the moon light

On that white fluffy cloud

The cloud is swaying gently in the air

Like a boat on smooth water

You can feel the movement as you gently float on the cloud

You are comfortable and relaxed

As you look around

You could see a dark blue sky

Other clouds, as they passed you

Bright stars are all around you

Some are so close you can almost touch them

You notice how peaceful the sky is

How calm it is and quiet

As you float higher and higher

You could notice your city

Lights into the windows

Take a moment to enjoy this beautiful sight

Rest in relax in the soft support of the cloud

Notice where your body is touching the cloud

How soft it feels

Notice how comfortable you are becoming

As you float through the sky

You feel safe, relaxed, and calm

Breathe in the clean fresh air

Take a deep breath in

Hold it for a moment

And now slowly exhale

You feel totally relaxed

Take another deep breath

And bring your attention to your head

Now exhale letting the tension leave your head

Your face

Your neck

Breathe in relaxation

Feeling your shoulders, arms and hands relaxing

Breathe out all the tension

As the air flew the weight of the tension out of you

You become lighter and lighter

Imagine you sinking deeper and deeper

Into the cloud

The cloud is all around you

Warm, soft, calming

Again, inhale slowly and deeply

As you exhale, feel the tension leaving your chest and stomach

Breathe in

Allowing your upper, middle and lower back to relax

Feel the tension leaving you as you release the breath

All the muscles of your back are light and relaxed

Again, inhale

Feeling the relaxation flowing through your hips, legs, feet

 And slowly breathe out

While stress, tension, and distractions are leaving you with the
air

Your body gets lighter and lighter

As you take another deep breath

Let all the muscles of your body release the tensions, relaxing fully

From head to toe

Breathe out, relaxing even further

Feel lightness in your body

Now you are feeling deeply relaxed and calm

You are very light

You are totally relaxed

Floating on the fluffy cloud

Feel the cloud supporting your whole body

It is a wonderful feeling

It is very safe

Very calming

Very relaxing

You are so relaxed

Floating on a cloud

Your cloud can take you wherever you wish

Higher, lower, side to side

Let your imagination free rein

Fly wherever you want to be

Continue floating relaxing

Enjoy the sights around you

(pause)

When you are ready

Allow your cloud to begin you back to earth

Right into your bedroom

The cloud slowly and gently places you on your bed

You are still feeling calm and relaxed

Bring your attention back to the room

Become aware of your surroundings

Now you may open your eyes

Still savoring the feeling of comfort and relax

Keeping that relaxation in your mind and body.

Have a good night

And follow your dreams!

Color Visualization
Color visualization can be an incredible procedure to enable you to loosen up, soothe pressure, and even nod off. Rather than concentrating on your on edge, a dreadful picture, mental exposure to colors enhances your capacity to concentrate on quieting and soothing pictures.

This calm shading visualization enables you to unwind wit representation by envisioning each shade of the rainbow. rainbow comprises of violet, indigo, blue, green, yellow, orange and blue colors. This meditation will depict each shading t enable you to unwind by contemplating on the hues.

Visualization can be especially compelling to unwind because enables you to concentrate your psyche on an envisione picture. This center is critical to reflection and unwinding by an large.

Take your position at the place of your meditation

Stay in a completely relaxed manner

Don't do anything immediately

Ground yourself first

Just stay completely relaxed for a few minutes

Get into a comfortable position

Keep your back straight

Ensure that your shoulders are also straight

Your back and neck should be in a straight line

Now, close your eyes

Find the best and most comfortable position

Try to feel your whole body

Notice if there is tension anywhere

If you feel any part tense, release the tension

Adjust your body to release the pressure

Focus on your breathing

Inhale from your nostril

Hold your breath for a few seconds

Exhale from your mouth

Breathe in

Hold

Gradually breathe out

Don't rush the process

Just notice how your breath goes in and out

Every breath that you take is bringing peace inside your body

Breathe in

Observe this inhalation carefully

Feel the sensation the air makes are your nostrils

Feel it expanding your chest

Hold the air for a few seconds

Now exhale

Remove all the air inside you

The air going out through your mouth is taking away all the negative energy from your body

You feel completely relaxed with each exhalation

Your stress goes out with this exhalation

Breathe in slowly

And hold

Relax while you exhale

Feel your body relaxing

Your jaw slackens and your teeth are not touching

Your eyelids feel overwhelming

Your shoulders drop a little lower

Your arms are peacefully lying down

Enable your physique to be loose, centered, and calm

Again, take a deep breath in

Hold it for few seconds

Slowly exhale

Notice how calm and regular your breathing is now

Continue breathing slowly through all the practice

Now in your imagination allow the rainbow colors to appear before you

You may envision items, light, or only a strong color

Imagine red of all shades

Envision the majority of the various tones of red

Cherries, bricks, roses, raspberries, red Ferrari, sunset, wine, red apples…

The red color is associated with excitement, danger, passion, energy, and action

Appreciate the red shades

Let the shading in your mind change to orange

Imagine the limitless shades of orange color

Pumpkins, oranges, fire, carrots, autumn, apricots…

Fill the whole visual field of your inner consciousness with the orange color

Orange represents creativity, adventure, enthusiasm, success, and balance

Appreciate the shading orange

Now picture the shading yellow

Let your creative mind find all the different shades of yellow

Enable yellow to fill your vision with lemons, chicks, bananas, sun, honey, sunflowers, gold, corn, pineapples…

Envision the unlimited tones of the shading yellow

It evokes feelings of happiness, optimism, positivity, and summer

Envision yourself encompassed with the quieting shading yellow

Appreciate the shading yellow

Presently find in your mind the shading green

Encircle yourself with green

Unending shades of green such as forest, leaves, limbs, grass, mint, cucumbers, frogs, green apples...

Drench yourself in the green color

Green represents growth, fertility, health, and generosity

Appreciate green color

Let the shading in your mind turned out to be blue

Fill your mind with the blue color

Unlimited tones of blue such as sky, water, cornflowers, jeans, blueberries...

Feel blue color from the lightest to the darkest, sky blue, tiffany blue, electric blue, azure, blue navy, space dark blue, and so on

Blue transmit stability, harmony, peace, calm and trust

Appreciate the blue color

Let the shading in your mind to become violet

Concentrate on the huge number of purples around you in the form of lavender, plums, brinjal, grapes, blackberries, viola flowers...

Envision violet filling your vision

Purple is connected to power, nobility, luxury, wisdom, and spirituality

Appreciate purple

Again, envision the colors, one at a time

Red

Orange

Yellow

Green

Blue

Violet

Envision yourself encompassed with the quieting shading violet

It is a calming color

A relaxing color

You are feeling comfortable and safe

There is no fear, anxiety, or stress

You are very calm and composed

You are feeling completely relaxed now

Stop controlling your breath

Become aware of your surroundings

Extend your muscles and open your eyes

Go to bed and have a peaceful dream!

For another, it's tedious and in this way somewhat entrancing Since you will likely end up feeling sleepy, this smidgen of self entrancing can help. Note that it's not in the typical sense, fo example, "you are getting tired". Or maybe, you're simpl accomplishing something dreary with your mind that will hav the impact of making you drowsy.

1

Remove mood killers or diminish the lights

Expel any clamor diversions from the room

2

Move into bed and close your eyes

3

Start with the number that you will check down from

A decent number to utilize is 100

4

Presently center on your relaxing

Attempt to keep your breathing as loose as could be allowed

Not taking in or out too forcefully

Envision that your breathing is quiet and relaxed...purifying

5

Each time you breathe out, you are going totally somewher around 1

6

Keep tallying down each breathed out breath until you arrive at zero

Envisioning that you are plunging further and more profound into your psyche at each tally

Different pictures and musings will most likely barge in while you're checking

This is normal

Simply let them unobtrusively aside by proceeding with the check

The speed at which you count must be regular

Neither too quick nor excessively moderate

7

Say to yourself:

Presently I'm going to begin tallying back beginning at 25

As I tell, I'll keep on diving into myself

Agreeably more profound into my relaxation

I will wind up sluggish and profoundly loose

Twenty-five

Twenty-four

Twenty-three

Twenty-two

Diving further and more profound at each check

Twenty-one

Twenty

Feeling lethargic yet at the same time wakeful

Nineteen

Eighteen

Seventeen

Skimming delicately down to each tally

Sixteen

Fifteen

Fourteen

Jumping, drowsy

Thirteen

Twelve

Eleven

Ten

Furthermore, the greater part accomplished, diving further and more profound into each check

Nine

Eight

Seven

Six

Five

Feeling extremely loose

Four

Making me increasingly loose and drowsy

Three

Two

One

Zero

Breathing wonderfully, gradually

Diving further and more profound with each breath

8

On the off chance that you arrive at zero and you are yet conscious

At that point rehash from 500 (or whichever number you picked in Step 3)

When you play out this tallying exercise, two things are occurring:

(a) You are utilizing the intensity of breathing as a method for keeping your brain in the present, as opposed to choosing not to move on or stressing over what's to come.

(b) The checking is utilized because it is an action that will occupy the psyche from other distracting considerations.

As you tally down, you'll see your mind start to meander

In the end your mind will totally float, and you'll nod off.

Visualize Your Next Day the Night Before

Pre-Sleep Visualization is a great tool to create a better tomorrow. Visualizing before bed is so powerful because while you are sleeping, your mind's subconscious process the last thing that you were thinking about. If you visualize your positive future before sleep, then you give yourself a head start, and you'll give yourself a good six to eight hours for it to start creating itself.

The last thing that was in your mind is something that you're going to be thinking about while you're sleeping. Unfortunately, most of us either think of things that went wrong that day or things that may go wrong the next day. Our subconscious mind absorbs all this and cultivates those thoughts for the whole night and then that negative thoughts become a reality in our life. So, it is crucial to visualize your next day in a positive way before going to bed.

Take place in your bed

Stay in completely relaxed manner

Don't do anything immediately

Just lie down completely relaxed for a few minutes

Now, gently close your eyes

Get into a comfortable position

Try to feel your whole body

Notice if there is tension anywhere

If you feel any part tense, release the tension

Adjust your body to release the pressure

Start by breathing normally

Become aware of your breath

Inhale through your nose

Exhale through your mouth

Take short inhalations

Hold your breath for a second

Exhale through your mouth longer

Breathe in

Slowly breathe out

Breathe in

Slowly breathe out

Again, breathe in

And slowly breathe out

Now focus on creating the next day exactly as you want

Visualize the entire day going exactly the way you want it to

Imagine as many details as you can

Be specific

Settle dates, times

Where are you?

Who's with you?

Visualize everyone being there when you call them

All of your priorities being handled

You are always on time

Completing every task with ease

Making every deal

How amazing does it feel?

Picture yourself victorious

Visualize yourself wellbeing, active and energized

Accomplishing more and more

Performing at your best in every situation

Feel the success of achieving your goals

What it feels like?

If you envision it, it will come

Your subconscious mind will work all night

On creating ways to make it all happen

Just as you have visualized it

When you are imagining your ideal day

It greatly increases your confidence and comfort level

You are also sending out your intention into the universe and to the other people

Get passionate about it before you go to sleep

Put a smile on your face

Go to sleep with positive energy

Chapter 7 Affirmations for Better and Smarter Sleep

Affirmations are phrases that usually start with "I" and include ideas that we can start to incorporate in our own minds. We often state affirmations to ourselves all day, but it can be hard to notice. They become ingrained in the way we think, and unfortunately, they are often negative affirmations.

These positive affirmations will make it easier to have healthier sleeping habits in your life. The more you can include these in your vocabulary, the easier it will become to see better sleep habits forming in your life.

Sleep Affirmations

To best practice using affirmations, say them to yourself as often as possible, especially when you are having negative thoughts. Even if you don't fully believe them at first, they will help you to eventually turn around your patterns of thinking.

Write them down and include notes throughout your house with the affirmations stated on them. Set alarms with these affirmations to help you remember to consistently include these patterns of thoughts into the way that you think. Below is a list of positive affirmations you can use to help improve your sleep.

Healthy Sleep Habits Affirmations

1. I am always looking for ways to improve my health.

2. I choose to incorporate habits in my life that will make everything else better as well.

3. I sleep when I am tired.

4. I wake up when I have had enough sleep.

5. I don't stare at my phone as I fall asleep.

6. I make sure to feel relaxed before going to bed.

7. When I have had enough sleep, everything else in my life will be better.

8. I have better focus when I am well-rested.

9. I have a better memory when I've had enough sleep.

10. It feels good to get the right amount of sleep and to take care of myself.

11. I feel better every day with each healthy habit I choose to include in my life.

12. I deserve to feel well-rested.

13. Getting the right amount of sleep is natural for me.

14. It is naturally healthy to ensure that I am centered on getting the best sleep possible.

15. I am always looking for ways to improve my sleep.

16. I do not allow myself to make bad decisions for my health when I know better.

17. I go to bed at the right time even if there is a distraction that keeps me up.

18. I make sure that I do not do anything that will prevent me from getting the right amount of sleep.

19. I allow myself to wind down before actually going to sleep.

20. My mind, body, and soul feel better when I have had the right amount of sleep.

Relaxing Affirmations

1. I feel more and more relaxed as I attempt to get the right amount of sleep.

2. I feel the relaxation throughout my mind.

3. I feel relaxed in every part of my body.

4. I am filled with peace.

5. I pour out serenity to those around me.

6. I am focused on becoming calmer and calmer.

7. I am not afraid of anything that might come my way.

8. I do not dwell on things that have already happened.

9. I release myself from the stress that I have already felt.

10. I do not restrict myself with fear over things that might be out of my control.

11. I know what is in and out of my control.

12 I fall asleep fast so that I can get the most amount of rest possible.

13. I do not fear stress; I know how to experience it at a healthy level.

14. I am excited about what tomorrow holds.

15. I do not fear the challenges I face.

16. I let the past stay in the past and do not let it drive my future.

17. I am present in this moment and focused on relaxing.

18. I relax throughout the day so that I can sleep better at night.

19. I sleep most peacefully when I release myself from my anxieties.

20. Peace and serenity are my normal states of being.

Deep Sleep Affirmations

1. I do not allow distractions that will keep me up all night.

2. I feel completely relaxed in my bed.

3. I surround myself with peace before I go to bed.

4. I fall asleep fast and make sure that I stay that way throughout the night.

5. I feel safe as I sleep, which helps me get a deeper rest.

6. I am able to fall back asleep even if I wake up at night.

7. I do not allow past restless nights to define how I will be sleeping now.

8. I make sure that everything around me promotes comfort so that I can stay focused on right now.

9. Sleep is a requirement for my health.

10. I am deserving of a deep and restful night's sleep.

11. I cut out habits that keep me from getting a deep sleep.

12. I separate myself from electronics in order to promote bette sleep.

13. I focus on sleeping the moment that I lay down for bed.

14. I always focus on my health so that I can get a deeper sleep

15. I clear my mind before bed so that I focus on nothing othe than drifting away.

16. I feel refreshed after making decisions for better relaxation

17. I manage my sleep in the healthiest ways possible.

18. Deep sleep gives me a deeper ability to process my thoughts

19. Stress does not consume me.

20. I am always focused on healthy sleeping.

Chapter 8 Meditation for a More Energized Morning

Sometimes, a part of waking up is doing so in a relaxed way. You might have to chill out a little bit before you will be able to fully wake yourself up!

If we go too fast all day, it can feel like we never fully get a break. This meditation is great for those who have a little bit of extra time in the morning to relax for a moment before heading off for the day. It can also be great for those who might want to listen to something as they eat breakfast, drink their morning coffee, or simply stay in bed for a few moments longer while becoming more energized.

This one was not designed to put you to sleep, but since it will still be a relaxing reading, you will want to ensure that you are in a safe location on the chance that you do drift off to sleep.

Waking Up Meditation

A new day has just begun, and now, it is time to start fresh. You are going to be starting out brand new with nothing from the day before holding you back.

To start your day off right, it is time to relax. Relaxing doesn't mean that you are going to be tired. This means that you are going to start your day with a clear head, a calm body, and a rested soul.

For this, you are going to want to do an exercise in which you make a fist, sticking your pinky and your thumb out with your right hand. Now, place your right pinky on your left nostril, pressing down. Now, breathe in through your right nostril.

Then, take your right thumb and press on your right nostril lifting your pinky up. Then release your air through your left nostril.

The point of this is to alternate the nostrils in which you breathe in and breathe out of. You will start to see how this can easily calm you down.

Do this again as we count. Breathe in for one, two, three, four and five. Breathe out for six, seven, eight, nine, and ten.

Once more, breathe in for ten, nine, eight, seven, six, and out for five, four, three, two, and one. Repeat this breathing exercise throughout the day when you need to calm down. Whenever you start to feel the panic rise at any time, try out this great exercise. It helps you focus on something while also ensuring that you are regulating your breathing.

Now, it is time to close your eyes and focus on becoming refreshed and new. You are going to start this day off right without anyone else distracting you. There aren't going to be things that keep you down. You are centered only on feeling as good as possible, all the time.

We are lucky to have a brand-new day each and every day. Although we might have to do the same things as we did the day before, it is time that we look at these things with a fresh mind. We are able to start over. We can be whoever we want to be today.

Release yourself from what happened before this moment. Remain proud of your accomplishments but forgive yourself for some of the decisions that you might have made. Keep your memories around, but only for good use. Remember the great times and learn from your mistakes. Don't ruminate on thoughts.

Prepare yourself to confront what you might need to confront today. Remember that you are strong and powerful, someone who is capable of absolutely anything. You are able to do all the things that you have dreamed of being able to do. No matter what you put your mind to, the results that you want will come.

Embrace the new day. Allow yourself to be open to what others might bring today as well. How will the people you know be different from yesterday? Can you be forgiving of others and mistakes that they might have made?

Breathe in positive vibes. Breathe out the fear that you have today.

Breathe in new experiences, breathe out your anxiety over what these experiences might bring.

Accept that even the things that might be challenging for you will also bring you new knowledge. Even things that seem scary or out of reach will give you new experiences you never thought possible. You will go through things beyond anything that you could easily imagine. You will always be tested on your strength, willpower, and resilience.

Take everything with pride. Assure yourself that you are capable of anything. Remember how brave you can be. Nothing is going to keep you afraid today. There are no things that you might confront that will bring you fear.

Breathe in the bravery that you need to conquer this day. Breathe out all of the feelings that you might not be able to do it. Remember how far you have come already.

You are not going to repeat what happened yesterday, or the day before, or the day before. Even if you did something great, today you will do even better.

You are going to make healthy choices throughout the day to help you feel like your best self. You will provide your body with nutrients, energy, and everything else it needs to function as well as it possibly can.

Remember to stay relaxed and stress-free throughout the day. When you free yourself from stress, you are letting go of all the things that might be holding you back. When you say "no" to anxiety, then you are granting yourself the chance to be happy and content with what you already have and with the things that currently surround you.

You are letting yourself go from the things that have held you back in the past. Your eyes are open now, and you see all that is needed to do in order to have the best day possible.

You are awake, alert, and energized. You are centered on breathing healthily and living happily.

You are not afraid of what is to come. You are entirely well-rested and have had all of the sleep that you need to be happy throughout the day.

You will have the chance to go to sleep later. You will have the ability to start over once again then tomorrow. There is nothing that is going to stop you from achieving greatness today.

As a final way to wake up, we are going to do one last quick hypnotic exercise. You are awake and alert now, but this will help you to feel even more energized so that you can have the best day possible. Each new day will be the best day because you will learn how to show gratitude, how to grow, and how to be entirely content.

Right now, continue to focus on your breathing. Keep your eyes open and hold your hand up so that you can snap it on command. With your eyes open, look up as high as you can without moving your head. This will result in your vision being slightly cut off by your eyelids.

Look up as high as you can using your eyes only, but not to the point that you are straining or hurting them. When we count down from three, snap your fingers on one and look in front of you. This will help quickly kick you awake and give you a little jolt of energy.

Keep looking up, higher and higher. On one, snap your fingers and look straight ahead. Three… Two…. One….

You are now awake, energized, and ready for the day.

Chapter 9 Meditation for Deeper and Healthier Sleep

One of the best ways to really become relaxed and find th peace needed for better sleep is through the use of visualization technique. For this, you will want to ensure tha you are in a completely relaxing and comfortable place. Thi reading will help you be more centered on the moment, alleviat anxiety, and wind down before bed.

Listen to it as you are falling asleep, whether it's at night or i you are simply taking a nap. Ensure the lighting is right an remove all other distractions that will keep you from becomin completely relaxed.

Meditation for a Full Night's Sleep

You are laying in a completely comfortable position right now Your body is well rested, and you are prepared to drift deepl into sleep. The deeper you sleep, the healthier you feel whe you wake up.

Your eyes are closed, and the only thing that you are responsibl for now is falling asleep. There isn't anything you should b worried about other than becoming well-rested. You are goin to be able to do this through this guided meditation into anothe world.

It will be the transition between your waking life and a plac where you are going to fall into a deep and heavy sleep. You ar becoming more and more relaxed, ready to fall into a trance-lik state where you can drift into a healthy sleep.

Start by counting down slowly. Use your breathing in fives in order to help you become more and more asleep.

Breathe in for ten, nine, eight, seven, six, and out for five, four, three, two, and one. Repeat this once more. Breathe in for ten, nine, eight, seven, six, and out for five, four, three, two, and one.

You are now more and more relaxed, more and more prepared for a night of deep and heavy sleep. You are drifting away, faster and faster, deeper and deeper, closer and closer to a heavy sleep. You see nothing as you let your mind wander.

You are not fantasizing about anything. You are not worried about what has happened today, or even farther back in your past. You are not afraid of what might be there going forward. You are not fearful of anything in the future that is causing you panic.

You are highly aware of this moment that everything will be OK. Nothing matters but your breathing and your relaxation. Everything in front of you is peaceful. You are filled with serenity and you exude calmness. You only think about what is happening in the present moment where you are becoming more and more at peace.

Your mind is blank. You see nothing but black. You are fading faster and faster, deeper and deeper, further and further. You are getting close to being completely relaxed, but right now, you are OK with sitting here peacefully.

You aren't rushing to sleep because you need to wind down before bed. You don't want to go to bed with anxious thoughts and have nightmares all night about the things that you are fearing. The only thing that you are concerning yourself with at this moment is getting nice and relaxed before it's time to start to sleep.

You see nothing in front of you other than a small white light That light becomes a bit bigger and bigger. As it grows, you start to see that you are inside a vehicle. You are laying on your bed, everything around you is still there. Only, when you look up you see that there is a large open window, with several computers and wheels out in front of you.

You realize that you are in a spaceship floating peacefully through the sky. It is on auto-pilot, and there is nothing that you have to worry about as you are floating up in this spaceship. You look out above you and see that the night sky is more gorgeous than you ever could have imagined.

All that surrounds you is nothing but beauty. There are bright stars twinkling against a black backdrop. You can make out some of the planets. They are all different than you would ever have imagined. Some are bright purple, others are blue. There are detailed swirls and stripes that you didn't know were there.

You relax and feel yourself floating up in this space. When you are here, everything seems so small. You still have problems back home on Earth, but they are so distant that they are almost not real. There are issues that make you feel as though the world is ending, but you see now that the entire universe is still doing fine, no matter what might be happening in your life. You are not concerned with any issues right now.

You are soaking up all that is around you. You are so far separated from Earth, and it's crazy to think about just how much space is out there for you to explore. You are relaxed, looking around. There are shooting stars all in the distance. There are floating rocks passing by your ship. You are floating around, feeling dreamier and dreamier.

You are passing over Earth again, getting close to going back home. You are going to be sent right back into your room, falling more heavily with each breath you take back into sleep. You are getting closer and closer to drifting away.

You pass over the earth and look down to see all of the beauty that exists. The green and blue swirl together, white clouds above that make such an interesting pattern. Everything below looks like a painting. It does not look real.

You get closer and closer, floating so delicately in your small space ship. The ride is not bumpy. It is not bothering you.

You are floating over the city now. You see random lights flicker on. It doesn't look like a map anymore like when you are so high above.

You are looking down and seeing that gentle lights still flash here and there, but for the most part, the city is winding down. Everyone is drifting faster and faster to sleep. You are getting closer and closer to your home.

You see that everything is peaceful below you. The sun will rise again, and tomorrow will start. For now, the only thing that you can do is prepare and rest for what might be to come.

You are more and more relaxed now, drifting further and further into sleep.

You are still focused on your breathing, it is becoming slower and slower. You are close to drifting away to sleep now.

When we reach one, you will drift off deep into sleep.

Twenty, nineteen, eighteen, seventeen, sixteen, fifteen, fourteen, thirteen, twelve, eleven, ten, nine, eight, seven, six, five, four, three, two, one.

Chapter 10 Meditation to Fall Asleep Instantly

This final meditation in this set is one that is going to help you fall asleep instantly. It is a quicker and shorter meditation that will take you through the visualization exercise.

This process makes it easier for your mindset to go from one where you might be thinking of specific things in your life to a place where you can get into a more dreamlike trance. You will be able to easily fall asleep and get that deep rest you need in order to conquer the day tomorrow. Again, ensure that you are in a comfortable place where you will be able to fall asleep for several hours at a time. This is best at night but if you plan on taking a rather long nap you could do this as well. Keep an open mind and focus on your breathing.

Meditation for a Deep and Quick Sleep

Sleep is incredibly important, but sometimes falling asleep can be difficult if we are not in the right mindset.

For this activity, we are going to take you through a visualization that will help ensure that you can get a deep sleep. It's important before falling asleep to relax your mind so that you can travel gently throughout your brain.

Start off by noticing your breath. Breathe in through your nose and out through your mouth. This is going to help calm you down so that you are able to breathe easier.

Begin by breathing in for five and out for five as we count down from twenty. Once we reach one, your mind will be completely clear. Each time a thought passes in, you will think of nothing.

You will have nothing in your sight, and you will only think with your mind.

Make sure that you are in a comfortable place where you can sink into the space around you. Let your body become heavy as it falls into the bed. Keep your eyes closed and see nothing in front of you but darkness.

Each time a thought comes in, keep pushing it away. Breathe in through your nose and out through your mouth.

Remember to breathe in for five and out for five. Keep an empty mind and be ready to travel through a journey that will take you to a restful place.

Twenty, nineteen, eighteen, seventeen, sixteen, fifteen, fourteen, thirteen, twelve, eleven, ten, nine, eight, seven, six, five, four, three, two, and one.

You see nothing in front of you, it is completely dark and you feel your body lifting gently up like a feather. You are light against the bed, and nothing is keeping you down. Continue to feel your body rise higher and higher. You are floating in space. There's black nothingness around you. You are gently drifting around.

You can see a few stars dotting the sky so far away, but for the most part, you see nothing. You feel yourself slowly moving through space. Your body is light and free, and nothing is keeping you strapped down. You're not afraid in this moment.

You are simply feeling easy and free. Breathe in and out, in and out.

You start to drift more towards a few planets, throughout your journey in space. You can really see now that you are up in the highest parts of the galaxy. You see out of the corner of your eye that you can actually catch a glimpse of Earth. You start gently floating towards it, having to put no effort in at all as your body is like a space rock floating through the stars.

Nothing is holding you down.

Nothing is violently pushing you either. Everything that you feel is a gentle and free emotion. You get closer and closer to Earth now and can see all the clouds that surround you. You start to move down, and you gently enter into the cloud area. Normally gravity would pull you down so fast, but right now you're just simply a gentle body drifting through the air. You get closer and closer to the land. You can see some birds here and there and a few cars and lights on the ground beneath you.

You pass all of this. Gently floating over a sleepy town.

Look down and let your mind explore what is it that you see down there. What is it that is in front of your eyes? What do you notice about this world around you as you continue to go closer and closer to home?

You are gently drifting throughout the sky. You can see trees beneath you. Now, if you reached your hand down, you'd even be able to gently feel a few leaves on the tops of the tallest trees. You don't do this now because you're just concerned with continuing to float through the sky. That's all that you really care about in this moment.

You're getting closer and closer and closer to home now, almost ready to fall asleep. You start to see that there is a lake.

You gently float down to the surface of the lake, and you land right in a boat. Your body is a little bit heavier now. You feel it relax into the bottom of the boat. Nothing around you is concerning you right now. You feel no stress or tension in any part of your body. You are simply floating through this space now.

The boat starts to gently drift on the lake. It is dark out now and you look up and see all the stars in the sky. All of this reminds you of the place that you were just a few moments ago. You start to drift closer and closer to sleep.

Do you feel as the tension leaves your body? You are peaceful throughout. You are not holding on to anything that causes you stress or anxiety. You are at ease in this moment. Everything feels good and you have no fear. You drift around in the water now for a little bit longer. You can see everything so clearly in this night sky. Just because it is dark does not mean that it's hard to see. The moon casts a beautiful glow over everything around you. You can feel the moon charging your skin. As you drift closer and closer to sleep, you feel almost nothing in your body now. You continue to focus on your breathing. You are safe, and you are at peace. You are calm, and you are relaxed. You feel incredible in this moment.

The boat starts to lift from the water. You feel as it gets higher above the water. You are even heavier now. Now you are completely glued to this comfortable surface as the boat starts to fly through the sky. You can look down and see that the city beneath you has drifted to sleep. You're getting closer and closer to home now. You can actually see your home beneath you. The boat gently takes you to your front door, and you float right in. No need to walk or climb stairs. You simply float in and straight to your bed.

You fall delicately into your bed with your head resting nicely on a pillow.

Here you are, in this moment, so peaceful and so relaxed. You are completely at ease. There's nothing that stresses you out or causes any anxiety or tension now. You are simply a body that is trying to fall asleep.

As we count down from 20, you will drift off to sleep. You will be in a very relaxed state where nothing stresses you out. You're not concerned with things that happened in the past, and you aren't going to stay up in fear of what might happen tomorrow, you are asleep. You are relaxed.

Breathe in and out. Breathe in and out.

Twenty, nineteen, eighteen, seventeen, sixteen, fifteen, fourteen, thirteen, twelve, eleven, ten, nine, eight, seven, six, five, four, three, two, and one.

Chapter 11 Implementation

IF and this is a big if; if you decide to take action and begin using these scripts; you will experience change. Your mind will get stronger. You will begin to feel unstoppable.

As you start your day feeling unstoppable, you may start to smile as heads turn to look at you. Your friends may even say you look different. Did you lose weight? Cut your hair? Just win the lottery? Only you will know why you are feeling so much better.

All this really means is that you have two simple choices to make, right now.

Choice #1: You can take this information and ignore it.

Choice #2: You can take this information and implement it into a daily routine.

"How often do I need to practice these scripts?"

You should look at self-hypnosis as exercise for your mind. Even though there are cases when a radical change can occur from a single hypnosis session; it is most likely that you will need a certain amount of reinforcement to undo years of bad programming.

If you can practice *one thirty-minute session in the morning upon waking and one thirty-minute session in the evening* prior to sleeping, you could expect to see a maximum change that would allow you to achieve a near miraculous change in your life in virtually any area you choose.

If you can do this three days per week, that will still help a lot. Once a week and you may continue to struggle; falling back into old habits and not really making any measurable progress. Consistency is the key to speed up your progress toward victory.

Next you need to know exactly how you are going to use these scripts. Ideally you will record them in your own voice at a slow even pace. Alternatively, you can have someone speak them to you, which you can in turn record for multiple playbacks in the future. And lastly you can simply read them to yourself.

You can probably guess that the first option will be the most effective and have the greatest impact on your subconscious mind. *Recording these scripts in your own voice at a slow steady pace will bring you tremendous results.* As you read, imagine that you will be speaking in a soothing monotone, almost like you are trying to put the listener to sleep. You will also want to match the tempo of some soft gentle music playing in the background, which brings us to the next point.

Avoid the temptation to speed up your speaking or to speak with emphasis; simply follow the script with a calm low voice; almost as if you are gently speaking to someone that is sleeping and you don't want them to wake up.

Ideally, as you are reading these scripts, you want to have soft gentle music playing in the background. Music has a way of opening up neural pathways and helps you to be more receptive to hypnotic suggestion. There are a ton of great soundtracks available on YouTube that you can use or you can purchase CD from your local music store.

The other simple option is to read your script and then overlay the soundtrack later with your selection of gentle music. Depending on the resources you have available to you, you will need to find a method to record yourself speaking the script out loud.

It is not sufficient to wake up in the morning and then try and read your script in bed or worse to simply try and read affirmations to yourself in your mind. This will not be as effective as listening to the scripts, you will likely just fall back asleep or your mind will drift off into different directions. You need to be fully awake and then find your dedicated relaxation spot. Ideally this will be a comfortable chair that allows you to recline to the point that you are able to rest your head and neck completely. A recliner style chair is of course ideal, but you can also use an office chair if the back is high enough to allow you to rest your head on the backrest and your feet are positioned comfortably in a resting position.

In your dedicated relaxation chair, you will play your recorded scripts in sessions of approximately thirty minutes. Once in the morning after waking and once in the evening before going to sleep.

This radically simple yet effective personal transformation system will work for you, even if you're overwhelmed, over stressed, and feel like you've been pulled in a thousand different directions. Maybe you've listened to hundreds of motivational tapes or attended seminars only to find that positive energy disappears by the time you returned home. Maybe you feel like you barely have enough hours in the day. Even if you feel as if you've tried absolutely everything!

Self-hypnosis is not a system of getting you pumped up and excited one minute only to leave you flat and depleted a short time later. This isn't a tactic that promises you'll get a mansion with a Ferrari in the driveway simply by thinking a bunch of positive thoughts without taking any action.

This system is based on years of dedicated research of experts in the fields of hypnosis, psychology, influence, persuasion, and personal empowerment. Many others have used these techniques to achieve greatness and now, starting today, their success can be your success. The strategies of the truly successful can now be easily duplicated, giving you the freedom to make decisions without agonizing delays, work at full mental power all day long for weeks and even months on end, eliminate anxiety and worry forever and never allow these toxic emotions to overpower you.

Keep other people from taking advantage of you and turn misfortune into opportunities. You'll be able to destroy objections and stop people from saying no and make it easy for them to say yes. Yes you'll even sharpen your ability to lead and influence others whether in private conversation or before a crowd of hundreds.

Now before we go one step further, I need to be 100% honest with you. If you're looking for yet another cheerleading session on motivation, something to pump you up for a short time while only to leave you deflated just a few days later , something you absolutely know is never going to work for you and it's only going to keep you frustrated in a vicious cycle of failure.

In short, there are no easy shortcuts for lifelong persona empowerment but following these powerful self-hypnosi techniques will propel you towards consistently achieving you desired goals and is truly as easy as it gets.

If you want to become your true, most authentic self, stop feeling stuck, stop feeling overwhelmed, stop procrastinating stop worrying about the future. Achieve your peak level of performance day in and day out. Say goodbye to the limiting beliefs, limiting patterns and bad programming that holds you back. Recode anxiety, anger and doubt into attitudes, beliefs and actions that you can use to serve you and fast-track you to a better, prosperous life.

If you want real-world, time-tested and proven techniques and strategies for really achieving your desired outcomes as quickly and easily as possible then this self-hypnosis program isn't just one solution for you - it's the best solution for you.

Please remember that these scripts are not intended to diagnose or treat any kind of medical condition; if you are unsure whether you need medical attention, please consult with a qualified hypnotherapist or medical doctor for direct help.

At this point, I should make a comment about the scripts; you will notice that the grammar of the scripts is unusual because they contain run-on sentences and many pauses. This is because the scripts are intended to be read in a continuous style of monotone to help in inducing the hypnotic state. If you see a word in bold or in all capital letters, it means to emphasize the word distinctly and slowly but not with a louder volume.

You will still benefit to a limited degree by just reading the scripts to yourself but remember that for maximum effectiveness; you really want to have these scripts recorded with soothing music in the background and then you can listen to them repeatedly at your leisure. And of course the scripts often instruct you to close your eyes so it is rather difficult to continue reading with your eyes closed! There is also a lot of similarity between the scripts, which is to be expected since they follow a similar process for implementing the hypnotic state.

So, without further delay, let's move on to the specific scripts for each area of powerful hypnotic programming.

Chapter 12 How to Do Self Hypnosis

It is time to learn how you can put yourself in a hypnotic state. Remember that what you are about to do is a process so never skip a step. Also, the effects will slowly change you and thus you may not notice the changes right away after just one session, you might though notice that you feel at least slightly refreshed, similar to how to feel once you wake up from a short nap. Give it some time and feel the measured change with every self hypnosis session that you do. Further, do not force yourself to enter in a trance right away; your subconscious will only fight you back no matter how your conscious mind tells it to do.

The following section will also be presented in bullet form and thus numbered for you to easily track which step you are in. Naturally, you need to be familiarized with the process first before you try it out in order to avoid the disruption of reading through a step again.

The Step By Step Process

You must have a clear goal for the session. Think about that and try to formulate a way to suggest to yourself to easily achieve this goal. Once you have the method to make it easier, create a statement that you can use to let you focus on that goal. For example, if you wish to become a better cook, then you must say "You are a better cook." Always say things how you want them, do not mention what you do not want.

Find a place you are comfortable in. A suitable location would be your bedroom since it is the comfort zone for most people, could also be your favorite spot in the house or somewhere outside where you'll have privacy. Just be sure that no one bothers you, let others know you need some time alone. Be totally honest on what you are about to do for them to understand the reason why you are doing so.

Decide on how long you wish to stay in trance. Setting a clear time limit will allow you to conserve the energy you need later to reinforce the suggestion you are about to say to yourself. A timer or app will help in this situation, be sure to set it to vibrate or at a low volume – as you want to slowly come out of your trance.

Calm down and then close your eyes. Keep a constant pace of breathing and slowly relax your entire body. Once you feel you are completely relaxed, start telling to yourself (in your mind) the statement you created in step one. While hearing this statement mentally, imagine yourself becoming a person in the statement. Repeat it over and over again while being continuing to relax your entire body. With each repetition the picture you see mentally must become clearer and clearer.

As much as possible, blot out any distraction your other sense might feel. It might take a while to master this step so do not be discouraged if you are unable to do so the first time you try it out. If you get distracted, just come back and focus on you intention, this is also the same technique used in self guided meditation.

Once you think you are able to reach the time limit you set in step three then tell yourself to open your eyes slowly. Continue the relaxed state and keep your phase of breathing. Then completely open your eyes and feel that you are out of the trance.

After you are able to completely get back to reality, start reinforcing your autosuggestion by doing a task related to the statement you created. In the example given, you might want to start out by making a sandwich or a simple meal.

1. Repeat the process in a regular schedule to amplify the phase of the effects. 1-2 sessions per day only when starting out, as you don't want to overload yourself, which could result in self sabotage.

As an added step, if you find being distracted while performing step four, you might want to try and count backward from ten to one each time you breathe. Likewise, to come back from trance in step six, count backward again to pull you completely out of the hypnosis if you are still unable to keep your concentration without the aid of counting in step four.

Again, these steps will not be able to show you abrupt results. The suggestion you gave yourself will gradually improve. Thus, constant practice must be present. Relax and let your subconscious mind drive your body with the new instructions you have just given it.

Chapter 13 Maximizing the Effects of Self Hypnosis

So, you have just learned one method of doing self-hypnosis there are many different methods that work. Now is the time to learn how to maximize its full effects. Maximization is technically not required for you to do. But doing so will allow you to feel and observe the change better.

Relax

Pressuring yourself to feel the effect right away will do you no good. The word relax was constantly repeated in the steps if you can recall. Likewise, even after the session, you must continue to relax yourself. Reinforcement also works best if you are in a state of mind that is capable of receiving information without distraction. Stress can also limit the effects of self-hypnosis so where possible avoid it, or don't let yourself get caught up in stresses. Relaxation can also help you in this part.

The Ripple on the Water

Notice that murky water will not allow you to see what is on the bottom of a pond. For you to see the bottom, you can either clean the pond completely which takes time or to try and use a stone to create a ripple. The ripple on the water's surface will give you a temporary view on how the pond will look like if the water is clean. Utilizing multiple ripples will push the dirt all the way to the side allowing you to clean the pond easier later. The same applies in self-hypnosis.

Doing multiple session as mentioned earlier will amplify the effect. But it does not mean that each session must have the same goal. You can change the statement you are using to create complementary effects. If we return to our example of becoming a good cook, the first statement you use can be "You are a good cook." Be sure this will be the most general goal. In the next session, you can try out telling yourself "You can create a delicious sandwich." Each goal then will give the previous one more reinforcement and thus will eventually lead to the first ever statement you used. Of course you can work on many facets of your life all through self hypnosis, different sessions will be needed for each area of life you want to change or enhance. Start slow and build up, take notice of the little things in life that you automatically do, especially those things that do not add any value to your life, these things, such as biting your nails, cracking your knuckles, having a smoke after dinner and many such other things, are usually all automatic subconscious learned behaviors & habits that we do without really thinking about it. If we took a moment to notice what we are doing several times a day you'll realize that more things you'd rather change about yourself. Which of course you can use the tool of self hypnosis.

Chapter 14 When You Can Expect to See Results

Since you are likely practicing self-hypnosis with the intention of getting some form of results from the experience, you may be wondering how soon you can expect to see the results. While the answer somewhat varies from person to person, there are some general clues you can consider which will help you determine when you can expect to see results in your own unique practice.

How Many Sessions Are Needed?

While many people wonder how many times they will need to use self-hypnosis to achieve their desired results, the reality is that there is actually no magic number that is all-inclusive for everyone. In fact, the number of sessions you need may change as you change what your focus is. For example, if you use self-hypnosis to destress, it may take several sessions. If you use self-hypnosis to quit smoking, it may take several more.

There are many considerations that factor into what results in you can expect to see and how many sessions are needed to get there. One includes how extensive the "problem" is. For example, if you have been smoking for several years and you have a strong addiction, you will likely need more hypnotherapy than someone who has only been smoking casually for a few years at most.

In general, the best way to see results from sessions is to be focusing on a few tasks at a time. While you should only set one intention per session, varying what intentions you focus on each session and then "cycling" back through previous intentions is a good way to ensure that you get the most out of your session.

110

Most "problems" are caused by a myriad of things. For example, a smoking addiction may be closely related to stress, which may be related to work and family life, and the stress there may even stem from childhood. As you can see, most "problems" have a stronghold in your life, stemming out into many areas. By targeting all of these during your various sessions and cycling through, you set the intention to heal EVERYTHING leading to your addictions, rather than just any single thing.

Most professional hypnotherapists claim that they cannot promise how many sessions it will take, but that the average person will see results beginning to take hold from anywhere between 1 to 6 sessions. It is important to understand that these sessions are being facilitated by a professional and that professionals are not actively involved in the hypnotic state so they can direct you in different ways than you can direct yourself. For that reason, you should recognize that it may take you several sessions to get to where you need to go. Fortunately, you are your own hypnotist in self-hypnosis, so as long as you take the time for you to facilitate your own session, you should be able to engage in your hypnotherapy practice as often as is required to see your desired results. Remember, the more deeply-rooted the problem is, the longer it will take to see results. You may begin to see basic results early on, but to truly overcome everything that is associated with your desire for change may take longer than it would with a professional hypnotherapist.

How Soon Can I Expect to See Results?

111

As with how many sessions you may need for your success, how soon you can expect to see results also varies somewhat from person to person, as well as from problem to problem. In general, most people will notice basic results early on, even as early as one single session. Again, it largely depends on how deeply rooted the problem is and how long it has been going on. The deeper the problem and the more issues you face as a result, the longer it will take for you to see results. You should notice, however, that with persistent action and intention, the results do not take terribly long to come around. If you remain intentional, schedule regular sessions for self-hypnosis, and ensure that you are fully entering a hypnotic state every single time, then it becomes significantly easier for you to see results sooner.

Generally, you will experience various results of your hypnotherapy session almost immediately after any given session, even the first one. However, these results may not be "complete" yet, so it is important that you do not waver and that you continue to practice your hypnotherapy on a regular basis until you experience complete relief.

In addition to specific results you are expecting to experience you will also experience other side-effects from your hypnotherapy session. These include things such as:

- Peace

- Relaxation

- Excitement

- Feeling "lighter"

- Calmness

- The world may seem "brighter" to your eyes

So while you may not instantly lose the weight you desire to lose, get a great new job, quit smoking without any more cravings, or otherwise experience your results right away, you will still get great side effects that help you recognize that the practice worked and that you are well on your way to becoming a healthier, happier version of yourself.

How Often Should I Do It to Maintain Its Effectiveness?
How often you need to maintain your self-hypnosis practice is generally fairly dependent on what the situation is. For example, if you are trying to overcome nail biting and you find that you have quit nail biting and have no desire to do this at any point in the future, there is a good chance that you do not need to use any reinforcement hypnotherapy sessions to keep your habit at bay. Instead, you can assume that you have overcome it and that you can move on. However, if you were to begin feeling inclined to bite your nails again or you noticed the habit had started again, or if you noticed your habit had merely switched and now you are doing a different form of nervous habit, then you would want to use reinforcement sessions to overcome this experience.

A general rule of thumb is that the stronger the habit or problem is, the more you need to set the intention to overcome it and therefore the more sessions you will need. Complete addictions, for example, may require several reinforcement sessions to help you get over your addiction and refrain from having any cravings that leave you feeling as though you want to begin your addiction once more. Habits, on the other hand, are less likely to require as much effort and therefore they are likely to be overcome in fewer sessions.

The best part of self-hypnosis is that you are completely capable of calling the shots. If you have worked steadily toward overcoming a habit, and then several weeks later you notice you have a craving or that the habit seems to sneak back in, you can go ahead and begin doing a self-hypnosis session as close to that experience as possible. Often, we can even find time to do it right away or within a few hours of the experience. Then, because it happened so quickly and we were able to stay on top of it, the habit will disappear once more with little struggle. Since you can call the shots and use this tool whenever you need it, it makes overcoming virtually anything from stress to addictions or even food cravings or a lack of motivation that causes you to struggle from losing weight. You can use it as often as you need and with any issue you need.

How Often Should I Schedule My Self-Hypnosis Sessions?
Knowing when to schedule your sessions is important. Like with most healing modalities, you need to leave a bit of time in between sessions to give yourself the opportunity to truly experience the healing that comes from each session. Otherwise, you may indirectly tell your subconscious mind that this practice is not reliable and therefore you will not gain the maximum benefits from your self-hypnosis sessions.

In general, you want to wait at least 12 hours between sessions on something that is particularly difficult, or 24 in between sessions on something lesser. If you experience complete relief, however, you will not need to worry about scheduling a reinforcement session afterward as there is no need for this extra session. Instead, simply go with the flow of your regular life and only call on this practice again if you feel that you are noticing complete relief was not, in fact, granted. Some people may feel completely relieved for the first few hours and then "come down" from that relief the first few times around. Do not worry about this happening. This does not mean your self-hypnosis practice is not working, it merely means that the habit has deeper roots and therefore requires more action and intentional hypnosis sessions to alleviate the problem entirely. Remember, cycle through everything that may be contributing to the problem and then come back around to the start so that you can eliminate everything that may be leading to you inadvertently reinforcing the issue in your own life. For example, if you want to lose weight but struggle to eat healthfully, you would want to focus on both weight loss itself, your struggle to eat healthfully, and anything that may be making it difficult for you to eat healthfully (such as stress).

Conclusion

The general conclusion about how much time is required to begin seeing results and when you will become effective is really one that cannot be answered easily. The amount of time you require to get your desired results will vary. It may take as little as a single session to overcome something if you were already willing to overcome it anyway and your desire was strong enough that it had already sunk into your subconscious on some degree and begun taking place. Alternatively, it may take several sessions over a span of several days or even several weeks to get the results you desire. As long as you stay committed and continue practicing self-hypnosis as often as needed, you should see great results from your practice.

Chapter 15 Practical Uses for Hypnosis

Hypnosis is a very versatile tool. Pretty much any issue that is rooted in thought processes can be fixed through hypnosis. There are also plenty of symptoms that can be relieved by tapping into the unconscious mind. When you are trying to figure out if hypnosis can help with a certain problem, there are two main needs:

1. Is this problem organic? If your goal is to find relief from a physical injury or illness, then you should see a doctor. With your doctor's approval, hypnotherapy can be helpful in some symptoms. It's important that you go to the doctor first.

2. Is it a mental illness? If it is, then you should go see a psychiatrist or psychologist first. Hypnotherapy isn't a cure-all for mental health; it's a tool to help change the habits and behaviors of mentally healthy people.

With that said, there are hundreds of practical uses for hypnosis. Some of the most common ones are:

Stress Management

This stress could relate to a job, relationship, or you're just overworked and underappreciated. Hypnosis can help you manage the source of your stress and prevent it from spoiling your life.

To start, most hypnotherapists will teach their clients some self-hypnosis as a way to help release pressure in an emergency for those times when things start to get overwhelming. Sleeping habits will also be looked at to help manage stress levels. If there are certain people that are aggravating the client, you shoul look at strategies for handling these challenges that th aggravating person is causing so that the client can break the ol patterns.

Student Hypnosis

Hypnosis for students can help them by aiding in their self confidence and their ability to focus better. This improve concentration while in school, better retention reduced anxiet on test, and a host of other benefits. Hypnosis can be helpful to all students, whether or not they are having any problems.

For the students that do have problems in school, there are lot of different things that hypnosis can help with. Hypnosis can b focused on test anxiety if that's the problem. The students ca learn how to relax during the tests to help focus their minds o the subject. For those who are smart, yet lack motivation, the can learn how to work smarter rather than harder by harnessin their subconscious. For a student who can easily learn th information but has a hard time recalling, they can learn how to unlock the file cabinet in their mind when they need to.

Smoking Cessation

Helping somebody quit smoking is quite exhilarating becaus you are saving somebody's life. But, the golden rule of hypnosi still has to be followed: You can't make a person quit smokin if they don't actually want to. If a person is truly interested i giving up smoking, hypnosis can be very effective. When using hypnosis for smoking cessation, you will:

- Figure out what will motivate you to remain as a nonsmoker

- Discuss what caused you to start smoking

- Go over the scientific information of the effects that smoke has on the body and fast the body is able to recover from smoke after you stop

- Use regression therapy to figure out the area of the mind that makes you continue to smoke and assign you the new task of staying smoke-free

- Make use of triggers and anchors to help you work through your cravings that come up during the early parts of the process

These are all big areas that hypnosis is used in, but there are plenty of others. Here are some more:

- Phobias and fears – This is great if somebody is afraid of the dentist, speaking to a group of people, and flying. Hypnosis can help you work through these fears.

- Unconscious habits – Negative self-talk and nail-biting can be resolved through hypnosis.

- Better sleep – If a person suffers from insomnia, hypnosis can help them get a full night's sleep.

- Headaches – If you get permission from your doctor, hypnosis can do an amazing job with chronic headaches that are caused by minor ailments, tension, or stress.

- Anger management – For the most part, people who have fits of rage suffer from a buildup of stress.
- Weight management
- Motivational coaching
- Self-hypnosis training

Even still, this is only scratching the surface of what you can do with hypnosis.

Chapter 16 Sleep and Physical Health

The reasons for insomnia may be mental, behavioral, physical or environmental. Even though it is easy to categorize causes, they blend deeply, making it difficult to single out any one reason. Yet, there are some important physical catalysts of insomnia that need immediate attention and solution.

Allergy Symptoms

Climatic or seasonal changes or heredity are a cause of insomnia. For example, respiratory problems like Asthma or difficulty in breathing due to pollen in the air or maybe an insignificant resistance to dust.

Allergies are volatile as they have a tendency to flare up to any extent.

Pain Related

One of the most common physical causes of insomnia whether mild or chronic, for example headache, neck pain, jaw pain, back pain, arthritis, muscular pain, weak constitution leading to frequent stomach spasms, etc.

Insomnia in Women

Hormonal changes during the premenstrual or postmenstrual cycle, late or early pregnancy, pre-menopause or post-menopause can result in physical discomfort. Women are lighter sleepers than men and these factors only add to their physical anxiety.

However, this nowhere proves men to be less prone to Insomnia.

Exercise and Nutrition

What you eat and drink has a direct impact on the quality of sleep. Intake of Caffeine and Alcohol has an adverse effect on sleep as these are stimulants. Lack of physical exercise leads to loss of vitality in the body, which in turn leads to physical exhaustion. This hinders a smooth sleep cycle.

Medication

Anti-Depressants are major culprits of Insomnia. Over the counter medication for minor medical problems like cold and cough is a cause of Insomnia. Heart medications, Asthma medications, Anti-Smoking medications are all the factors that kill the environment for a perfect sleep.

Other Obstruction

Thyroid, Digestive Inflammation, Chronic Fatigue syndrome, Acid Reflux, Bowl Syndrome, Gastric infections etc.

Physical Effects of sleep deprivation

Since the body loses vigor and vitality due to insomnia, it has a direct impact on your physical well-being and may turn a mild case of insomnia into chronic

1. Dark Circles and Eye Bags: Since you leave the body wanting more sleep, it tells on the areas around the eyes which demand rest from strain.

2. Irregular pulse

3. Increased risk of Coronary Heart diseases

4. Risk of prostate cancer due to late working hours

5. High blood pressure

6. Strokes

7. Diabetes

8. Slow motor skills affecting our driving competence, work performance etc.

9. Major genetic changes due to prolonged and persistent sleep loss e.g. obesity (due to hampered Glucose metabolism) and hypertension

10. Major dip in sex drive due to depleted energy levels

11. Accelerates aging process -tiredness that surfaces as wrinkles on the face

12. Increased risk of death due to excessive burden on our vital organs

13. Slow healing process (wounds take much longer to heal due to weak immune system)

14. Over indulgence in heavy medication may be treated as cause and effect both. Use of medicines to recover lost sleep leads to a vicious circle where the savior itself becomes the destroyer

Every problem has a solution; you just need to find it, cementing it with self-discipline, determination and composure.

Chapter 17 Time for Bed

Eat some gelatin or take glycine

It's usually best to stay clear of desserts after dinner since sweet can give you sugar rush making you feel pumped and more alert But gelatin is an exception. Gelatin is made up of glycine and proline, amino acids that you might not consume in adequate amounts since they are found in the organs, bones, and fibrous tissues of animals. These amino acids are important since they help your body boost immunity, control weight, and have proper hair, skin, and nail growth. One way to get these amino acids in your system is to consume gelatin. Aside from being a wonderful health supplement, gelatin can also help you sleep with ease. Studies show that people who eat gelatin before bedtime are able to sleep better and report less daytime drowsiness. Take note that we're not referring to those sugar and preservative filled gelatin with artificial coloring. It's best to go with the unflavored ones.

Write a list or meditate

Your body needs to shift into sleep mode by relaxing so it is best to spend the last hour before bedtime doing calming activities. Meditating before going to bed can also help your sleeping pattern. It is best to do the sort of mediation that helps you relax your muscles. This type of meditation makes you tense up then relax your different muscles to promote an overall state of relaxation. Relaxing promotes better sleep as it helps with the transition between the wakefulness state and the drowsiness state. Writing a list of the things you aim to accomplish tomorrow also helps you to worry less as you have prepared a time or schedule of how to handle all your tasks for the next day. Some even suggest doing journaling, as it helps you release all your thoughts about the day that you just had. Clearing your mind from the stress of the day helps you relax. This way, you won't find yourself lying awake in bed because you're worrying over something. It also helps if you keep clocks out of sight. Knowing what time it just makes you conscious of the fact that you are losing sleep and before you know it, you're counting the hours pass by.

Take some Magnesium

Magnesium usually gives your body an energy boost and that same energy indirectly helps your body to be in a restful state after the boost. This is because magnesium helps your body wind down in preparation for sleep as it helps your muscles relax, giving your body a neuroprotective vibe, something that will not only help you fall asleep but will also keep you asleep. Some people find that rubbing their body with magnesium lotion or oil can give them vivid dreams. You know this works when you feel some stings as you rub. Although some would actually feel the opposite and will have a hard time sleeping after a magnesium rub. It really depends on your body system.

Block all forms of light in your room

When you eliminate all sources of light in your bedroom, your body system automatically shuts down in the darkness. Even the light emitting from the hallway under your doors is enough to distract you from sleeping. Try placing some rags or a thick mat under your door for total darkness. Use blinds on your windows instead of curtains so that you can block out light from streaming in your bedroom through your windows easily Remember that the tiniest bit of light—even the soft glow from your alarm clock—can interfere with your sleep. You can also simply use an eye mask to trick your brain that you are in total darkness if you have family members or roommates who are not ready to turn of all the lights yet in your home.

Read something fictional

And when I say read, I do not mean ebooks but paperbacks. Do not pick novels that are exciting or with storylines that will not allow you to put the book down because you will only get to the point where you want to read "just one more chapter" and before you know it, it's daybreak and you didn't get any sleep at all. Go for old-english books or old literature; even some fantasy is good if it doesn't keep your mind adventuring. Pausing to analyze some sentences or thoughts can easily make you fall asleep. Some suggest spiritual books can also help you forget about your worries as they usually aim to uplift the spirit and will put your mind to peace during bedtime.

Take a tablespoon of honey right before bed

Take note that I am not referring to sweetened, artificial honey but to raw honey. According to studies, taking a tablespoon of honey keeps your liver glycogen full thus improving sleep quality. Studies claim that raw honey contains the ideal ratio of glucose to fructose for supporting the liver. Our liver works overtime while we sleep. Honey makes sure that the liver will have enough liver glycogen to keep it running throughout the day and night, restoring and detoxing your other body functions. Aside from great sleep, you can also benefit from numerous health benefits that your system can get from taking a tablespoon of honey before bedtime.

Use white or brown noise to block unwanted sounds

There's a reason why bats, being nocturnal animals, prefer to stay in caves for their sleep during the day. This is to achieve an environment that blocks the noise from outside, allowing them to sleep well. You can also avoid unwanted noise by using earplugs while you sleep or using a white noise appliance. If you share your bedroom with someone and that someone happens to be a big snorer, purchase earplugs or get some headset on and listen to nature tracks. Have you noticed that it's easier to sleep or take a nap when it's raining? This is because the sound of falling rain is calming and relaxing. You can listen to nature sounds such as rain, running water, birds tweeting, the sounds of a forest or an ocean while going to sleep. Listening to such tracks can help you ease up and relax and before you know it, you'd be drifting off to dreamland.

Chapter 18 Behind the Scenes

So what is it that makes us sleep at night and automatically wake up after a set number of hours (if you've ever encountered that)? To understand the influence sleep has over your mind & body, you must understand the mechanism that triggers it first.

I won't get you warry with the details and keep it as simple as possible. The first of these entities is known as Homeostasis. This is more of a process through which the body maintains its current balance when it comes to blood pressure, internal temperature, etc. The amount of sleep one encounters every night is also controlled by homeostasis.

From the time a person wakes up, homeostatic drive for sleep triggers up. The drive keeps building up until its late evening when it is at it's peak. This homeostatic drive is controlled by a hormone called adenosine. These levels rise continuously as long as the person's awake and "tell" the body of the growing need for sleep. During sleep, the adenosine levels drop and keep on dropping until they are at a threshold level at which point they disrupt the sleeping process.

Sleep deprivation occurs whenever there is too much accumulation of sleep debt and it becomes impossible for the body to go on without repaying it. For instance, when a person stays up all night, his body will demand that the lost hours be made up in some manner, by napping or by longer sleep cycles. It has been found that even the loss of a single hour of sleep at night can build up for days and result in negative performance at home or work.

Homeostasis was the first of the two factors. The next one is the body's Circadian rhythms. These are cyclic changes and there's a pretty good chance you've heard of these if you've ever gone through sleeping issues. The cyclic changes are much like fluctuations in body temperature or hormone levels and are controlled by our internal "body clock" ironically known as circadian clock. The clock is synchronized with the external environment and is unlike our typical real world ones. The strongest agent that can affect this circadian clock is light. Light and darkness have a profound effect on this clock and slowly it adapts to the conditions it is put in.

So putting it all together, the homeostatic system makes us sleepier with the passage of time whereas the circadian system tries to keep us awake as long as we're in contact with light. But this is the best case scenario. If your body's internal clock is synchronized with the day-night cycle, then you'll have no problems with your sleep and you'll always wake up with a great mood and motivation. However, when you push your body to the limits either intentionally or unintentionally the balance starts to deteriorate and the clock no longer works as it should. Anyone who has traveled cross-country or worked at night would be quite familiar with the set back the body goes through with respect to sleep.

As stated before, the circadian rhythms are the body's internal way of telling us to wake up and sleep. We can definitely go against them and when we do the first thing that happens is diminishing of our mental & physical state. Jet lag is the most infamous symptom of disruption in the circadian clock.

But that isn't the end of it all. There are several factors that are still playing their part as you sleep. What are they? Find out next.

Chapter 19 Lifestyle Changes

Along with stress-relief and a healthy diet, your sleeping schedule can be optimized through a couple of lifestyle changes. These are in no way major changes and can easily be a part of your daily routine, requiring a small amount of dedication from your side. They are as follows:

Transform your bed:

Your bed should be a place where you can unfold and free of any kind of distractions or clutter that can impact your sleep adversely. Get rid of all unnecessary junk that is either on or around your bed. Laptop, trailing wires, fancy cushions, etc. are just a few examples. Try your best to get a mattress that suits your back; this is especially true for people over 40 as the wrong mattress may cause back pain as well.

Here are a few ways to control bedroom noise:

- Use earplugs,

- Install double-parred windows and decorate with heavy curtains,

- Use a fan or appliance that produces steady "white noise". White noise devices are specifically available in the market to eliminate all other interferences.

Reduce lighting in the room:

In order to get the best possible quality of sleep, try your best to eliminate all sources of light in your room. Turn of all types of devices that have LEDs etched in them and make sure the curtains properly cover the windows if you plan on sleeping late

Researchers at Max Planck Institute have found through a se of experiments that when people were kept in an isolated environment and told to sleep, their circadian clock responded in a much better pattern. Changes in the light intensity entering the room revealed that the patterns changed significantly as the intensity increased. The light had an inverse relation with the release of melatonin, the sleep inducing hormone.

Eliminate Blue Light:

Light is a spectrum that consists of 7 colors. There are a range of frequencies (energy) that are emitted from any luminous source. Out of all these wavelengths, red light has the least energy while blue light has the most. Even you would've noticed that using laptop or smartphone just before going to bed disrupts sleep patterns. Slowly your sleepiness fades away and before you know it you've spent half of the night surfing the internet.

The main reason behind this is the emission of blue light that can reduce melatonin secretion dramatically, down to 39%. So even if you plan on having a small night-time bulb, try to avoid one that gives off blue light.

Turn down the thermostat:

The onset of sleep is directly influenced by the room and body temperature. Researchers at Cornell University, New York found out that even though a person's body temperature doesn't have that much of a hold on his/her sleep hygiene, it does greatly affect the onset of sleep. Turning down the thermostat to a mildly warm temperature can accelerate the entire process.

Set regular bed timings:

This is one of the best methods to ensure better sleep hygiene. Try your best to go to bed at the same time every day. Sure, that is something impossible in this day and age but try keeping the overflow limited to 1 – 2 hours. By doing so you'll be able to adjust your circadian clock. In a few days you'll notice that you'll automatically wake up at the same time every day, sometimes without any alarm

Taking a nap:

Between 7 AM and 9 AM your body is highly energetic; every task put ahead of you feels like a new challenge, one that you can accomplish easily. But when the clock strikes 3, the energy levels drop to very low levels. You'll find it very hard to concentrate on one particular entity and you'll be out of focus every few minutes.

If you use this "low energy" time for sleep, then you can greatly replenish your body's resources. Don't wait until all your body's energy has been drained out. Instead, nap for half an hour between 1 PM and 4 PM. This will recharge you and get you stimulated about the task ahead of you.

If for some reason you have a lot of sleep deficit, you can fill it up by sleeping during this time period.

Avoid sleeping medications:

Having a uniform circadian clock is your best bet against sleep deprivation. If you try to mold it to your will every time you face a hurdle, then after a couple of nights you'll find it very hard to sleep without external factors. Sleeping pills are commonly used in every household due to the fast paced nature of this century. However, they can disrupt the circadian cycle and offset the mind-body balance. In fact, the use of sleeping pills can increase your chances of suffering from episodes of insomnia.

Chapter 20 Health Implications of Improper Sleep

Daily life activities can sometimes make people forget about the importance of a good night's sleep and proper rest. The truth is, every living being with a nervous system needs to sleep, and we are not an exception. Several studies indicate that people who sleep less than six hours every night are at more risk of dying, and only after one night of not sleeping properly cerebral tissue is lost.

So, you get the picture now? A good night's sleep is not only important; it is vital. Let's go through some of the negative effects of not sleeping properly or not sleeping enough.

Effects of Not Sleeping

Hunger and anxiety: lack of sleep provokes a tendency to ingest more calories, carbohydrates, and is associated with junk food cravings.

Increases accident risk: this is really a no-brainer; it's proven that people who don't sleep properly are at more risk of been involved in a car accident. The ocular coordination effects are the ones that play an important part in this.

Less attractive: bags under the eyes, tired look and premature skin aging are some of the effects of not sleeping properly. The hormone that gives elasticity to the skin and prevents wrinkles is released during the night, so sleep has a lot to do with you getting dates, or not getting any.

More chances to get the flu: defense mechanisms in your body are affected by the lack of sleep.

Loss of cerebral tissue: this is due to how the brain overloads with the lack of sleep affecting the nervous system.

Overly emotional: sleep, emotions, and behaviors share complicated mix of chemicals in the brain, so the lack of sleep makes your brain work harder and the nervous system is affected by this.

Memory problems: tiredness does not allow the brain to process information correctly, and this accumulates during the whole day. The brain is incapable of holding information and memory is not precise.

Difficulty focusing and concentrating: tiredness and sleepiness impede anyone trying to focus; this is simple. The brain doesn't get enough blood and it can't function at a high level.

Augments risk of embolism: the lack of sleep can put your body in a constant state of alert, and this augments the production of hormones that cause stress and tension, provoking an increase in your blood pressure.

Increases risk of suffering from obesity: this is also due to hormones like ghrelin and leptin, which work against you when you don't get enough sleep. *Here's a great book in leptin resistance*

Increases risk of suffering from cancer: several studies associate the lack of sleep with colon and breast cancer.

Diabetes: the body's reaction to not sleeping is similar to what happens when diabetes is just starting. When there's insulin resistance the sugar levels in the body elevate and cause organ failure.

Cardiac problems: lack of sleep elevates blood pressure and this can provoke artery obstruction and cardiac failure.

Affects fertility: less concentration of sperm in the semen is what provokes this.

Lack of sleep affects genes: interruption of sleep or lack of sleep affects more than seven hundred genes, and for this the risk of suffering from diseases like cancer, diabetes, and many others increases.

Lack of sleep is also associated with anxiety, depression, diminution of libido, mood swings, bad temper, and the propensity of many chronic diseases. Now that you know all that can happen if you don't rest properly I bet you'll pay more attention to your biological clock and the needs of your body.

Sleeping Disorders

Sleep is like an indicator of your health in general. Healthy people tend to sleep well, but if you have sleeping issues, this can be an indicator of an underlying problem. There are many things such as stress, caffeine, cigarettes, lack of exercise, etc. that can cause sleeping problems. But if you recurrently have trouble sleeping at night, then maybe there's something else. We'll discuss some of the most common sleeping disorders so you can check if you might be dealing with a sleeping problem.

Insomnia

Insomnia is one of the most common sleeping disorders. Many people complain they don't sleep enough or that their sleep was simply not satisfactory. This can be due to many things like the bed not being comfortable, noises, high temperature, irregular routines, lack of physical exercise, eating too much before you go to bed, alcohol, cigarettes, or caffeine beverages such as coffee and tea. However, this sometimes can be caused by emotional problems, difficulties in daily life, stress, and depression.

Insomnia Symptoms

- *Difficulty falling asleep*
- *Waking up in the middle of the night and being unable to fall back asleep again*
- *Waking up several times during the night*
- *Sleepiness and tiredness during the day*

Sleep Apnea

Sleep apnea is also a common sleeping disorder. Apnea happens when your breathing stops momentarily during sleep because your upper airways get blocked. This interrupts your breathing and so your sleep also gets interrupted several times during the night. You might not remember these episodes, but the next day you will feel very tired. Sleep apnea can be moderate or pretty serious, and it can be caused by being overweight, pillows, a soft bed, among other things.

Sleep Apnea Symptoms

- *Loud snoring, usually chronic*
- *Pauses in breathing during sleep*
- *Choking, panting, difficulty breathing during sleep*
- *Feeling tired and without energy during the day even after sleeping for long hours*

- *Waking up with headaches, dry throat, nasal congestion, or chest pain*

Restless Leg Syndrome

Restless Leg Syndrome causes an irresistible desire to move the legs. People who suffer from this syndrome feel uncomfortable when they are in bed. Some people describe it as a tingling, crawling sensation. As with other sleeping disorders, alcohol, caffeine, and cigarettes can worsen the symptoms.

Advanced Sleep Phase Syndrome

Advanced Sleep Phase Syndrome is when people are unable to stay awake in periods where they are supposed to be active, so they sleep soon and early, but wake up in the middle of the night and can't fall back asleep. This syndrome is more common among older people.

Delayed Sleep Phase Syndrome

Delayed Sleep Phase Syndrome is a lot more frequent than Advanced Sleep Phase Syndrome, described above. It's characterized by difficulty sleeping. People who suffer from this syndrome sleep later than usual and have difficulty waking up in the morning. This can cause serious problems because these people's more active hours are past midnight. This can cause problems in work, school, or morning activities. This syndrome develops mainly between the ages of 16 and 18, as well as during the twenties. It's strange to see it develop in the thirties or later in life.

Nightmares

Nightmares are common, and I dare to say that everyone has suffered from nightmares at least once in their lifetime. But, what is not common is to suffer from nightmares every day. Food, stress, or emotional problems can unchain these terrible night experiences.

Bruxism

Bruxism is a sleep disorder that appears in the second stage of sleep and is characterized by lateral mandibular movements that cause intense friction between the upper and lower teeth. It's nocturnal teeth grinding, and it can provoke severe teeth damage and facial pain.

Any of these sleeping disorders, caused by stress or alterations in the circadian rhythm can provoke tiredness, irritability, digestive upsets, and other symptoms that can be worrying and very annoying. There are many things you can do to help your body sleep better and give your brain and your body some rest. If the problems persist, please visit your physician.

Chapter 21 Lifestyle & Sleep

A healthy lifestyle does not only influence your overall health, but also favors your sleep. Several studies indicate that people who make good lifestyle choices enjoy good health and sleep more profoundly.

There are habits that have positive effects in every stage of your sleep. Many of these habits or lifestyle choices, such as diet, environment, etc. are a matter of common sense, but many people tend to overlook them and, as a result, suffer from insomnia or other sleeping disorders.

Let's go through some of these habits that can help you clean up your sleep, and please consider that you have to be consistent to get good results.

Alcohol And Stimulants

You have to be really careful with the ingestion of stimulants. Caffeine is a good example: you can have a cup or two during the day, but if you drink many cups your sleep will be affected.

Nicotine is a stimulant drug that also interferes with your sleep. Symptoms of night privation can interrupt your most pleasant dreams. Besides, cigarettes are just bad for you!

Alcohol acts in a very peculiar way in your body: at first it induces sleep, but then it will interrupt it. Only one cup can translate into waking up many times during the night and nightmares. If you are going to drink, try to do it at least four or five hours before you go to bed, just as with coffee.

Exercise

Exercise not only helps your overall health, but is vital to get good night sleep. This is something you have to incorporate int your daily routine.

Even though exercise is beneficial for your health and you sleep, the time of the day you work out is important. People tha are in a good physical state should avoid exercising at least si hours before going to bed.

Exercising in the morning will benefit your sleep, but exercisin, in the afternoon or at a time that's close to your bedtime, ca: cause alterations in your sleep. A sedentary life, irregular o limited physical activity can also provoke insomnia or slee disturbances. So get it moving and work out a bit!

Stress Management

Stress is one of the most common things that trigger insomnia and there's a logical explanation for this. When your body i under stress, your brain responds, activating your nervou system, and when this happens your breathing and heart rat accelerates and your muscles receive huge amounts of oxygen As you can imagine, with all this happening inside you, sleep cai turn into mission impossible. It's important you learn how t manage stress and how to keep calm to be able to rest properl every night. In the next chapter we'll go through som techniques that will help you relax and work in your stres levels.

Night Routines

To enjoy pleasant sleep that can fulfill its purpose and recharge your batteries, a night routine that induces relaxation and sleep is necessary.

For example, setting a schedule to go to bed every night is beneficial. Your body gets used to schedules, this means you will get used to sleeping at the same time every night.

A good routine could be having a healthy dinner, then a relaxing shower, and while you do this, disconnect yourself from work and everything else. Then put on comfortable clothes, read a book and go to bed and sleep like a baby. Do this every day, exactly the same way and in the same schedule, your body will get used to it and your sleep will improve without a doubt.

Weight

If you have a few extra pounds, try to get rid of them. Being overweight can cause sleep apnea and interruptions in your sleep.

Sleeping Pills

I would like to finish this chapter by giving you some information about sleeping pills. Many people are desperate, but aren't really aware of the effects and consequences.

Sleeping pills have been used for a long time to help people who suffer from insomnia and other sleeping disorders. In actuality, we know that pills are not the answer. They are toxic and can provoke many serious side effects. In other words, they can make you feel miserable. Sleeping pills can cause tiredness, irritability, and they lose their effectiveness pretty quickly, meaning you will have to augment the dose every time, and that is unhealthy. There are many things you can try before using sleeping pills, so you should leave these at the side.

Lifestyle influences your sleep a lot! Good lifestyle choices are beneficial for your entire body, not only your sleep. Be smart about what you do, what you eat and stay healthy in every aspect of your life.

Chapter 22 Natural and Alternative Treatments for Quality Rest

Give Yourself Acupressure

Stemmed from the process of acupuncture, acupressure is a technique that is classified as alternative medicine that involves bringing flows of energy to specific areas of the body. Pressing on specific points and giving them pressure allows your body to restore balance within these various areas throughout the entire body. It helps you to regulate the body, mind, and spirit. Chinese medical history has shown many success stories regarding this practice when it came to getting a better night of sleep as well.

- Begin between your eyebrows. There is a depression in that location, right above the nose. Gently apply pressure to that area for a total of 1 minute.
- Now find the depression between your first and second toes located on the top of the foot and press there for a few minutes until you feel a slightly dull ache.
- Look at your foot as if it is split up into 3 sections, starting at the tips of the toes and ending at your heel. Find the area that makes up the one-third of your foot that is behind the tips of the toes and press there for a few minutes.
- Now apply just enough pressure to make for a nice massage behind your ears and massage behind them for 1 minute.

Foods that Help You Sleep

There are various items you can consume throughout the day that can aid greatly in helping you gain the deep, recharging type of sleep you so desperately crave. All these items have within them natural remedies that aid and promote a better quality of sleep.

- *Walnuts* – Walnuts contain a grand source of the sleep-enhancing amino acid tryptophan, which aids in the production of serotonin and melatonin. It has also been found that these nuts contain their own amounts of melatonin as well.
- *Almonds* – Almonds are rich with a mineral that is necessary to get a good quality of sleep, magnesium. There are many studies to prove the negative effects that a lack of magnesium within the body can have, one of them being the inability to stay asleep once drifting into slumber.
- *Cheese and Crackers* – There is an old tale that warm milk makes you sleepy. This is true, but dairy products overall aid in sleeping. Calcium, which is found in almost all these items, assists in the brain's utilization of tryptophan. Calcium is also responsible in the regulation of muscle movements.
- *Lettuce* – Having a healthy salad with your dinner can help in the speeding up of the bedtime process. Lettuce contains a sedative property known as lactucarium which affects the brain similarly to opium.
- *Pretzels* – Yummy items like corn chips and pretzels contain a high glycemic index. With their consumption comes a dramatic spike in blood sugars

which results in shortened times it takes you to drift to sleep.

- *Tuna* – Salmon, halibut, and tuna are fish that contain high levels of vitamin B6, which you need for your body to properly make melatonin and serotonin. Other foods with B6 are pistachios and raw garlic.

- *Rice* – Rice not only helps you to feel full longer but is also high in the glycemic index, so it helps slash down the time it takes to fall asleep. Specifically, consuming jasmine rice has been proven to help its consumers get shut-eye much faster.

- *Cherry Juice* – Drinking a nice cold glass of cherry juice before bed helps with the natural boost of melatonin levels. There have been studies that improve the quality of sleep in insomnia patients who started to regularly drink cherry juice 1-2 hours before bed. The more tart the flavor, the better!

- *Cereal* – A neat bowl of your favorite flakes can aid in sleep. This good bedtime snack has two things needed for great sleep: carbohydrates and calcium.

- *Chamomile Tea* – This kind of tea is known as a stress buster. Drinking a cup of chamomile tea before bed increases glycine, a bodily chemical that aids in nerve and muscle relaxation. It also acts as a mild sedative.

- *Passion Fruit Tea* – Drinking a cup of this tea at least 1 hour before bedtime helps those who consume it to sleep much more soundly throughout the nighttime. Harman alkaloid, a chemical that is found within the passion fruit flower, is said to make changes to your nervous system when consumed, resulting in making you tired.

- *Honey* – Known as a natural sugar, honey has man different benefits. Regarding getting better sleep, raises insulin levels that let tryptophan enter th brain. Mix a teaspoon of honey with chamomile te for a great, natural sleep aid.

- *Kale* – Leafy veggies like kale are full of calciun which boosts our body's ability to utilize tryptopha that promotes the production of melatonin. Mustar greens and spinach are other great options!

- *Lobster and Shrimp* – Here is a great reason to indulg in your favorite seafood! All kinds of crustaceans ar loaded with sources of tryptophan, which can brin on much easier sleep.

- *Hummus* – Chickpeas, which are the main ingredient of hummus, are a great source of tryptophan. So, ea some hummus on delicious whole grain crackers as good bedtime snack or before you indulge yourself i an afternoon catnap.

- *Elk*- This game meat has twice the amount o tryptophan than meats such as turkey, which mean you have the potential to fall asleep not too long afte consumption.

Chapter 23 Termination

Now that you are ready to fall asleep, I want you to send your focus to how heavy and warm your body feels. Feel how warm your hands are and allow that feeling to spread through your whole body.

Take a few moments to notice how heavy your eyelids are. As you continue to breathe gently, they become heavier and heavier. It feels wonderful to rest your eyes as they remain relaxed and closed. All of the tension you had earlier has left and drifted away without a care in the world. Each breath you take allows the tension to slip through your fingers and your toes. All that you have left at this moment is total relaxation.

Now, allow your mind to drift away. There is no need to focus or think in these final moments before you drift off to sleep. Your mind is relaxed. Your body is relaxed. Your whole body feels warm, soft, and totally relaxed.

Your body is sinking down...down...deeper and deeper...focus on your breath as you slip into a comfortable sleep...

One...

Two...

Three...

Four...

I want you to keep counting on your own now. Try to focus on the numbers as they pass through your mind. If you lose count, start at one again. All you need to do is keep counting. Allow your thoughts to drift and tun back to the numbers. It become a lot of effort because you are so tired. It is becoming harde and harder to focus. Your mind keeps drifting away as you fal asleep.

Gently bring your thoughts back and begin counting again. Witl each breath, try to count the numbers again.

One...

Two...

Three...

Four...

You are finding it hard to focus. All of the numbers are blending together. You are much too sleepy to count at this moment. You are drifting deeper, hardly able to keep your thoughts straight.

It is okay. Now, just relax and continue to breathe gently. There is no need to count any longer. Allow your mind to drift off tc sleep. Surrender to the heaviness of sleep. Allow yourself to slip back into your happy place. This place is quiet and peaceful. You feel safe and relaxed.

Now, your body begins to feel like a feather. Your body floats gently toward sleep. You drift back and forth, down further and further toward sleep. Soon, you will rest peacefully in your safe place. You are so sleepy and gently drifting.

Now, I am going to count from number one to the number five. There is no need to count along with me. When I say the number five, you will drift off into a full night of sleep. Ready?

One…you are filled with total relaxation. Allow yourself to fall into this comfortable sleep.

Two…after this session, every muscle, and nerve in your body is completely relaxed. Your limbs are loose and limp. You feel wonderful from the top of your head to the tip of your toes. You are ready to fall asleep in any moment now.

Three…you are feeling perfect in every way possible. You feel perfect physically. You have worked through this session to help your body heal itself.

You are feeling perfect mentally. You have worked through your issues and let go of the stress you have been holding onto. You are feeling calm and relaxed. You allow yourself to be happy and completely serene at this moment.

Four…you are almost completely asleep right now. Any moment, you will drift off and sleep through the whole night.

You are completely relaxed. Now, you will allow yourself to fall asleep. You will experience a wonderful and deep sleep like you never have before in your life.

In the morning, you will wake up at the correct time. You will wake up feeling full of energy, relaxed, and fully rested. By getting a full night of sleep, you will be setting yourself up for success tomorrow. You will love yourself and practice your new positive thoughts. Remember to breathe through the stress and try to be your most authentic self.

Breathe in...breathe out...when I say the number five...you will slip out of hypnosis and sleep.

Have wonderful dreams and enjoy the journey.

Conclusion

It is not difficult to hypnotize someone immediately, but your success needs to be confident in yourself.

In a few easy steps, hypnosis can be applied to anyone. Next, ensure that your environment is conducive to your subject being hypnotized. This means dimming the lights and making sure that there are no distractions, perhaps lighting some fragrant candles. Get your subject comfortable by gradually breathing into your nose and expanding out of your mouth.

Then they get rid of all emotions, worries, or doubts by assigning each of them a color, and then eject them as they breathe in and out. Now ask the person to imagine a liquid that fills them from the feet to the head, and they will feel relaxed and comfortable when this happens. An idea, a thought, or even an action can now be suggested.

This is known as the hypnotic proposal. Visualization usually involves recognizing the wrong aspects of custom and then positive results when your custom is being dumped and when your subject feels far better.

After the person is allowed to stay in this "happy place," it's time to return. Hypnosis is helpful for people with sleep disorders, especially sleep hypnosis.

Sleep hypnosis may lead to managing a variety of slee disturbances. Some sleep disorders respond well to slee hypnosis, such as bed weather, sleep insomnia, or sleepwalking

Bed wetting affects people of all ages. Sleep hypnosis may lea to the identification and resolution of the issue. Sleeplessnes also reacts well.

This sleep disorder can be caused by psychological disturbance anxiety, or medication. Therapists can relieve stress and calr fear in nightmares, which is the cause of these awful dreams.

Sleepwalking, also recognized as sleepwalking, takes place at an age. It usually happens during deep sleep for the human.

While self-hypnosis may help an individual with minor slee deprivation, a professional should better diagnose and trea short-term and long-term disorders.

Sleep hypnosis fits with other therapies, such as counseling, medications, or a sleep diary.

CPSIA information can be obtained
at www.ICGtesting.com
Printed in the USA
LVHW051157220221
679611LV00009B/378